Practically Healthy

Practically Healthy

Step-By-Step Guide to Better Health

SPECIAL EDITION

Dr. Turshá R. Hamilton

To order additional copies of this book, contact:

Dr. Turshá Hamilton
www.DrTursha.com
info@DrTursha.com

ISBN:	**0692205357**
ISBN-13	**978-0692205358**

CONTENTS

CONTENTS

DEDICATION

This book is dedicated to all of you that have a true desire for more energy, better health, and a longer, more vibrant life but don't know where to start or how to continue.

I hope this information serves to help you obtain the best health that you can imagine, and then some!

DISCLAIMER

This book was written with the knowledge, education, experience, and opinions of the author. It is to be used as a guide to help you help your body heal itself. In that regard, the contents of this book are intended for educational purposes only. This is merely a guide. It is not meant to prevent, diagnose, treat or cure.

This book is not meant to be a substitute or replacement for medical advice, care or treatment by your health care practitioner. It is sold with the understanding that the author is not rendering medical, health, dietary, or exercise advice or services.

Your Naturopath, Primary Care Physician, or other health care practitioners should be consulted prior to adopting any suggestions described in this book.

The author and publishers specifically disclaims any and all liability, loss or risk, personal or otherwise, that may result from use and implementation of the contents of this book.

"A wise man should consider that health is the greatest of human blessings, and learn how, by his own thought, to derive benefit from his illness"

"The natural healing force within each of us is the greatest force in getting well"

- Hippocrates, Father of Modern Medicine

FORWARD

The information in *Practically Healthy* is designed to help you move beyond your physical and psychological constraints to achieving good health, even if that means challenging what you think you know. We've been totally misled on a number of things that directly affect our health. Dr. Turshá Hamilton reveals the myth then tells you the truth.

In her witty, conversational style, Dr. Turshá Hamilton dispels the myth that diet soda is better or "healthier" than regular soda. Many people believe that diet soda helps with weight loss but you will learn in *Practically Healthy* that diet soda does not help with weight loss. It actually contributes to weight gain, and it's better to drink regular soda than diet!

Many people believe that you should have a bowel movement only as often as you do. The truth is that you should have a bowel movement at least once a day, as Dr. Turshá Hamilton humorously explains in the chapter entitled, "Empty your Trash." She also tells you other functions of your digestive tract that will amaze you.

The feeling of hunger you get may just be your body's way to telling you that you're thirsty and need to drink some water.

A lot of people believe that the food we eat is the same as the food our parents and grandparents ate, but it's not; Dr. Hamilton shines the light of truth on the food that's available today, revealing that much of it is highly processed and lower in nutrition than the food our elders ate back in the day. She craftily uses a car analogy to demonstrate why we need to eat good food, not just food that tastes good.

We currently live in an age where many, if not most, of the people we know are living with chronic conditions and taking prescription and/or over the counter medications. It's so wide spread that we see commercials on television and whole pages in magazines advertising for prescription drugs. Nearly two-thirds of the U.S. population is obese and over-weight, and only about one-third of the population is at normal weight. Diabetes has reached epidemic proportions. Bariatric surgery is the new weight-loss miracle. Antibiotics, once called the "magic bullet," are losing their magical powers as we see more and more drug-resistant bacteria popping up. Food includes items developed in laboratories that have 70 ingredients or more. Much of the produce is heavily sprayed with pesticides and/or contains genetically modified organisms (GMO). Children are acquiring diseases historically seen only in the adult population and are being treated with drugs that are designed for adults. Many doctors are prescribing drugs for the side effects of the drugs that were prescribed for the illnesses. Everyone knows someone who has died of cancer. I can go on at the risk of growing tedious.

No wonder so many people believe that chronic illness is inevitable, exemplified by the old justification for unhealthy indulgences, "I gotta die of something." What's wrong with dying of old age? What can we do NOW to avoid the prescription LATER? Dr. Turshá Hamilton is an expert at treating chronic disease, but more importantly, she's an expert at prevention. As the old saying goes, "An once of prevention is better than a pound of cure."

Practically Healthy is like a choose-your-own-adventure style of health book with step-by-step instructions to guide you through the particular aspect of illness prevention and health promotion you'd like to explore. No need to feel guilty about not reading the book straight through if that's not for you because it's not designed to be read that way. It's designed for you to choose the topic that you'd like to improve and start there; the health topics are organized by chapter.

Dr. Turshá is one of the best givers of funny, practical advice. As a physician myself, it's hard not to second-guess advice from someone that's not me, but I trust Dr. Turshá Hamilton to give me reliable advice on any number of things. Dr. Hamilton and I are both licensed Naturopathic physicians trained at the same medical school. We're not just colleagues but great friends, which is another reason I take her advice. After having known this wonderful lady for close to 10 years, I can definitely say that in this book she's giving us the same practical advice that she would follow herself.

You have every reason to get started on your illness prevention, health promotion journey. If you really want to improve your health, do it! There's a scene in Star Wars V: The Empire Strikes Back that wonderfully illustrates the necessary approach to becoming *Practically Healthy*. Yoda is teaching Luke Skywalker to use the Force. Yoda says, "You must unlearn what you have learned." Luke Skywalker says, "I'll try." Yoda responds with, "No. Try not. Do... or do not. There is no try." Make the decision and just do something. Dr. Hamilton has said to me on a number of occasions, "either you'll do it or you won't."

-- Dr. Ayesha Worsham

PREFACE

Your body – your temple – is AMAZING!! It is a brilliantly intricate and complex machine. It is wonderfully resilient and is fighting every day to keep you balanced and alive!!

This is what I believe. This is what I know. I mean, think about it. When you cut yourself, doesn't your body work very hard to heal the wound? And of course, you know that if you clean and protect the wound properly, it can heal completely without a scar. The rest of your body is exactly the same way. If you clean it, protect it and give it the right conditions, you can heal just about anything.

That's the reason why I wrote this book. My goal as Naturopathic Primary Care Physician, is to help you achieve and maintain the highest level of health and vitality possible. The way to do this? Remove the "obstacles to cure," those things that impede proper healing. Once those are removed, you give the body the building blocks it needs to heal and repair. You are then on your way to becoming completely healthy... without a 'scar.'

I believe this book will give you the tools you need to create the thoughts, actions, habits, and traditions that will promote optimal health. The suggestions are practical. They are easy to incorporate into a busy, hectic life. Once you get used to one suggestion you can add another, then another. Next thing you know you'll look around and you'll be healthy... *Practically Healthy.* And that's what we are working for!!

All my years of seeing patients, lecturing crowds, teaching courses, and hosting radio shows, I've learned that the most successful changes in health come from those that make modifications in ways that fit into their lives and are consistent. No excuses. No whining. No giving up.

Just decide on the changes and do it… do it often. Simple. Easy. Practical!

User's guide:

This book is not a weight loss guide. It's not a new diet plan. It doesn't tell you how to quit smoking or help you prepare to run the Boston Marathon. That's not the reason the book was written. The book was written as a guide to help you build better habits in different areas of your life in order to build better health. The best way to use this book is to read chapters 1, 2 and 3 thoroughly and straight through. These chapters are intended to be your foundation for making healthy changes. Use them to understand what needs to be done and help you decide what areas you want to improve. You can also use them to help you plan your journey, discover your goals and prepare mentally for what is to come. With successful planning, you are much more likely to have the results that you are trying to obtain. From there, read each of the other chapters in the order you'd like and as often as you like.

This is by no means how you must do it, but in my opinion, starting there will give you the best outcome. Any way you decide to do it, be sure to give yourself time and remember to love yourself through the process.

Dr. Turshá Hamilton
Naturopathic Primary Care Physician

ACKNOWLEDGEMENTS

Thank you to my many patients, those who attended my lectures, and those that connected with me on FB, Twitter, and email. Your presence, your attentiveness, and your questions were, and are, valuable learning tools for me. I appreciate the trust you've given me.

To my family and friends: I thank you for allowing me to be myself, and all that it entails. Thank you for loving me and being there for me whenever and however I needed you.

To Dr. Ayesha Worsham: Thank you, "Roomie" for being the awesome friend, teacher, and colleague that you are. You are a beautiful, honest, loving, quirky soul. Thank you for never losing yourself no matter what roadblocks come your way.

To Vickie Thomas: Thank you for being a great friend, student, teacher, and sister. I appreciate you trusting me enough to work with me. I thank you for allowing me to be part of your healing journey. I look forward to watching you continue to blossom while you become a beacon of light, possibility and encouragement for others to follow.

To Brother Billie King: If it were not for you, I'd still not have this project completed. Thank you!! I appreciate your drive and determination. I look forward to EPIC things!!

I'd like to thank the friends, fellow authors that have encouraged me to write. As Authors, you provided me with examples of intelligence, tenacity and creativity. As friends, you would push me to do what I was supposed to do. Rhoda Lawson, Isha Cogborn, Harold "HB" Branch, Jae Henderson, and Shon Hyneman: Thank you all for leading the way for me and others that watch you do what you do so well.

Geveryl Robinson: Over the years you've been an amazing friend. I've admired your drive, creativity, and fearlessness. Thank you for all that you have done in your own life. You've been a reminder to me of endless possibilities and how to roll with the punches (and laugh at them in the meantime). Thank you also for being a SUPERB editor!! I appreciate you being patient with me through this process, even with all the awesome things you have going on in your own life and career. Many blessings to you. I look forward to seeing how your next ventures will unfold and shine!

To Lisa Perla: who knew what sharing a kind word with the person sitting next to me on the plane would lead to? Thank you SOOO very much for being willing to review my book and share your expert, unbiased opinions and recommendations! Thank you for your comments and encouragement and I wish you all the best in the world... and beyond!

To Mommy and Daddy: Thank you for always, <u>ALWAYS</u> supporting me. You always encouraged me to never quit. You supported my dreams, even as a little kid, and never let me lose sight of what I was supposed to do. Thank you both for being great examples of what an upstanding, loving, sensible, intelligent and caring adult is supposed to be. I am who I am because you are who you are!!

To everyone else that has walked with me through this journey, THANK YOU! Know that I really appreciate you and I do not take you for granted.

Turshá Hamilton, N.D.   www.DrTursha.com

CHAPTER 1

Let's Begin

୪ ଌ

"I'm not going for easy, I'm just going for possible... and what's in front of me right now is possible" – Sarah Murnaghan, an 11 year old, 2 time double lung transplant patient with cystic fibrosis.

It's an undeniable truth that the human body is a complex and amazing creation. The way we move, the way we develop, the way we communicate and learn are all very intricate. What's even more spectacular is the way we heal, the way we are resilient, and the way we grow. All three are such beautiful things, and as more scientific and technological advances are made, the more beautiful and fascinating the journey to understanding the amazing complexities of understanding our bodies becomes. So, before I delve into just how complex our bodies can be, let me begin with the basics.

In Naturopathic Medicine there are 6 basic tenets:

1. *Vis Medicatrix Naturae:* The healing power of nature. This is the idea that everything in nature, if given the right conditions (nutrients, cleanliness, time) will heal itself.
2. *Tolle Causam:* Treat the cause. Another great tenet. *Tolle Causam* is the idea that although symptoms can be treated as needed to make the patient comfortable, it is not until the cause of the malady is treated that the reversal of the condition and curing/healing the person can occur.

3. *Tolle Totem:* Treat the whole person. Now, each person is a whole being, and every part is interconnected. So, instead of looking at individuals as the sum of different parts (brain, spine, digestive system, lungs, etc.), looking at them as a total package and considering everything in a larger picture is more effective.

4. *Docére:* Doctor as Teacher. The physician has the charge of educating the patient, teaching the patient about what is happening, how to help the body heal itself, and how to prevent disease as best as the patient can. *Docére* creates patient empowerment, and empowerment is strength.

5. *Prévenir:* Prevention. Prevention is the best way to get and stay healthy.

6. *Primum non nocere:* First do no harm. Basically, employing the most effective methods of treatment that will do the least amount of damage to a body, will allow the healing process to move forward.

So, there you have it. Now, in case you are wondering why I am writing this book, my purpose is very simple: all of the above. As a physician and teacher, I want to empower you to prevent as much pain, sickness and disease as possible. My goal is to use the most holistic, least harmful and invasive methods possible to give you the tools needed so that your body can have the optimal conditions to heal itself. Once you have those tools, you will be able to live a longer, stronger, happier, and more vibrant life. And how do I accomplish my goal? Well, by giving you a broad spectrum of methods that you can use to help you become the whole, healed, vital person that you were meant to be. Hence, the reason for this book.

Practically Healthy, as its name implies, is a manual, a guide to help make improved health a practical part of your life. Health should be easy. Wellness should come naturally. The easier it is for you to incorporate healthy habits, the healthier you will become with less and less effort. That's not to say that becoming a healthy you will always be easy, but what it does mean is that you will become stronger, and the task won't be quite as difficult.

As you start to change your thoughts and actions to move you toward better health, always remember to give yourself permission to take your time to heal. Give yourself room to make mistakes. Love yourself through the process. Forgive yourself for what you've done in the past. Know that you can start where you are. And most of all, stay focused through it all, because this is how you see the greatest results.

Listen, I know making changes can be difficult. Change can often feel like an uphill battle as you break tradition and foster new habits, but it doesn't have to be. And yes, the changes will take time, but as time management guru Peter Turla once said, "It's better to do the right thing slowly than the wrong thing quickly." The changes don't need to be radical. What they do need to be is consistent. No matter what you do, continue to do it as often as possible.

Eventually, you will be doing different things automatically because the changes will have become second nature. This is how healthy habits are formed. This is where good health begins. Once you form good habits, you are on your way becoming *Practically Healthy*!

Now, before you start jumping around to the different chapters in this book, make sure you read chapters 2 and 3 thoroughly. As stated in the "User's guide" (found in the preface), your foundation is important. Knowing why it is important to make changes, planning for those changes, and then doing the associated mental work will make your Journey to Wellness much easier and the changes you make more permanent!

CHAPTER 2

Roadmap to Success

Ⳑ ⳍ

By failing to prepare, you are preparing to fail - Ben Franklin

"How Much Change is Enough?" You may wonder how many changes you need to make in order to achieve the health goals you are looking for. Well, those thoughts are valid, but the answer is a tad more complicated.

The short answer is, "I don't know. It depends." Let me explain. There is no one-size-fits-all answer to wondering how many changes need to be made, because everyone is different. The health challenges you face are all dependent upon several factors: age, genetics, past environment, and stress level to name a few. How much determination you have, how many changes you can make at one time, how long you can maintain those changes, your support system, and choosing the right modifications at the right time also play a role in how quickly you can get to your destination.

Let me give you an example. If someone were to ask you, "How long would it take to drive from Jacksonville, FL to Los Angeles, CA?" Well, if you were to look it up, you would find that the quickest route from one to the other is I-10 West which is 2,460 miles long. Now, if you were to drive all 2,460 miles only stopping for gas and to use the restroom, it would probably take you just under 2 days. 2 days travel is a rough guesstimate, due to the factors that might determine the true timeframe, such as the type of vehicle being driven, the rate of speed, and the number of people going on the trip who may or may not be able to help you drive, etc. I mean, you may decide to visit a friend in Mobile, Alabama. You might then decide that after your stop in Alabama, it might be a perfect time to stop in New Orleans for a few days to enjoy Mardi Gras or Jazz Fest. Maybe you get discouraged because a third of your trip will be going through Texas and it seems like it will never end (but since we all love Texas, that can never be the case, right??!!) Then there's traffic, weather, etc. There are so many things that can slow you down from getting to your final destination in the original timeframe.

Just like that road trip, your health journey takes planning, preparing, determination, time, patience, and a roadmap to help guide you to your final goal. If you can remember to stay on task no matter what detours and obstacles may come along, then you can reach your final destination.

Now that you understand all the variables, pull out a sheet of paper and a pen because there are a few things I want you to jot down to get you started.

STEP 1: Write down your ultimate goals. Do you want to lose 30 pounds? 300 pounds? Reverse Type 2 diabetes (because it IS possible!!)? Lower your cholesterol? Have acne-free skin? Reduce or eliminate allergies? Run a marathon in under 4 hours? Whatever your goals, write them down. It doesn't matter how many or how farfetched they are, just write. Now, once you've written down all your goals, take a look at yourself in a mirror and reflect on your health. After you have reflected, both literally and figuratively, go back to your list and decide which of those on your list is most important, then next important and so on. Number them so that you can have a visual of your plan ranked most to least important.

STEP 2: Decide when you would like to (realistically) reach each of these goals. If this task is too daunting for your entire list, just start with the top one or two. Remember to create a timeframe that you can actually achieve. Let's try not to make goals so unattainable that you will get discouraged early on in the process. Don't discourage yourself before you even get started.

Now that you've created that timeframe, what is half that? Use this as an example: if you want to lose 100 lbs. in a year, then half of that is 50 lbs. in 6 months. Take half that – 25lbs. in 3 months. If we kept this up and broke it down into bite-sized portions then you'd lose roughly 8lbs a month: 2lbs each week. Losing 2 lbs. per week is completely doable (and safe)!!!

STEP 3: Pick a start date for each goal on your list. You can start them all on the same day, stagger them by a week, or stagger them by a month. It's up to you. Remember that this is YOUR roadmap to success. No one can create your map for you but you.

STEP 4: Prepare. Now that you know what your goals are, have a realistic timeframe to work in, have a plan and a start date, it's time to properly prepare yourself. Do you need to go grocery shopping? Do you need to get rid of all the "junk food" you have hidden in those cabinets and secret places in your home, office or man cave? Should you get a few reusable water bottles to keep you on track? Maybe you need to get some new walking shoes, or a journal to keep by the bed. Whatever you need to do, begin to prepare now so that you don't have any obstacles once your start dates arrives.

You also want to get yourself mentally prepared for what lies ahead. Get excited!! Get Pumped!! Get motivated!! Let all your fear move to the side. Feed off the fear in small, motivating bites. Use it to make you even more determined to reach your goals. Do like athletes do at pep rallies and get HYPED before the big game!

Step 5: Re-evaluate the people around you. Are there negative people in your life? If so, begin to limit your contact with them as much as you can. Begin to find and surround yourself with positive, like-minded people that will encourage and support you through every phase of your journey to better health. You can also take note of how you respond to those negative people when they are being discouraging or less than supportive. Is your response also something that you need to work on? If so, add it to the list and keep it moving! Keep this quote in mind as you weed out the negative and plant the positive:

I may not be able to change my situation or a person, but I can change how I respond to them!

CHAPTER 3

Change Your Seat,
Change Your Life
☪ ☾

"Nothing can stop the man with the right mental attitude from achieving his goal; nothing on earth can help the man with the wrong mental attitude…" Thomas Jefferson

In Naturopathic medical school Dr. Michael Smith taught our business classes. During these classes he would make us change where we sat from time to time. If you were ever a student, then you know that once you find a seat that you like, or that you just get comfortable with, you don't change it very often (or ever) because it's your seat. You get complacent. You get attached.

When Dr. Smith made us change, none of us really liked it very much. We thought he was crazy for making us do it (at least I did, I can't really speak for the others). It was a hassle to have to pick up everything and move it somewhere else (not really, but it felt like it). Then we had to get resettled. Get re-acquainted with the students that were now our new neighbors. There were only a few of us, so getting reacquainted wasn't very hard; it just wasn't what we wanted to do.

Then one day, Dr. Smith asked us why it was important that we changed our seat. Of course, the first thing that came to my mind was something like "There's no reason, you just felt like making us move." But once he started to explain, it really began to make sense to me. By changing our seats, we changed our perspective in the class. We had to look at him, the overhead, and our classmates from a different vantage point. We were not able to get too comfortable and complacent because things were going to change soon. We had to be flexible. We also had to learn to handle change and the idea that things would change often, especially our seat in class.

As he discussed this concept further, I realized how much broader this concept was. Not getting too "settled" could be applied to every aspect of life. How you dress, your route to school or work, how you react to that guy that cut you off in traffic. No matter what the situation, there is always another perspective waiting to be gained. And changing the way you see a situation can make all the difference in the world. And now, even though changing seats was something I was not comfortable with at first that exercise is now something that I try to do as often as possible. I even have the students in my classes do it on occasion.

Dr. Smith's exercise reminded me of another point. No matter what, I had to go to class! I couldn't change my seat to, say, one that was in the movie theater for instance. If I didn't go to class, I would not be able to obtain my larger goal: Graduation → licensure → DOCTOR! So in that regard, my situation couldn't change.

The lesson in this case taught me that you can't always change or control the situation you are in (at least not without more radical, negative consequences sometimes), but you can modify how you react in that situation. By doing so, your perspective can have a major impact on your outcome.

As I mentioned before, this concept of change can be applied to every aspect of your life. By actually focusing on your ideas and beliefs, how they play out in your life, where they came from, and what results they've gotten you to this point, you can better see which ones have served you well and which thoughts need to be changed immediately! Some of them, once realized, will be a no brainer. You'll be able to immediately see what needs to be done and how you can take steps to make the necessary changes. A few of these will be easy to spot but a bit more difficult to work on, and that's ok. Realizing that change is needed and taking your time to find a solution is still moving in the direction of resolution.

There will be a few other thoughts/ideas/habits that are hard to see and hard to navigate. Some may be downright painful at times. During those times, it is probably best to find some support to help you work through the difficulties. Whether that support comes from a psychologist, a therapist, a counselor, a hypnotist, or your minister, the important thing is to seek the help and support from someone outside your normal circle of friends.

Keep in mind that all true and lasting changes- physical, mental, emotional or spiritual- start in your mind. They all have to begin with your recognizing and acknowledging that there is something in you that needs to be adjusted or modified in order for you to move to the next level of success. Acknowledgment is the first step on the road to your final destination.

Also keep in mind that overcoming mental obstacles is usually the most difficult part. Going back to analyze how you think about something, where those thoughts and beliefs stem from, why you act and react the way you do and then working on replacing your old thoughts with productive thoughts that are goal and dream directed, takes a lot of doing. However, as long as you stay focused on your goal and remain positive, it won't matter what may come along that will try to negate how you feel, or even who may come along to say negative things.

This is your journey and you should always be in control of it. You can always bring your positive friends and family along for the ride. And, you can even teach them some of the things you are learning along the way. You can do things like preparing different teas for them, cooking a healthy vegan meal for them, taking them for a walk, or involving them in your newest activity. You can even demonstrate breathing exercises or teach them to create affirmations. There are numerous ways to bring people on the journey with you. Just keep in mind that just like it took you a while to come around to where you are, it may take them a while as well. Don't expect them to change just because you did (I had to learn that one the hard way). Also, don't expect those you love to "get it" just because you did. The reality is that they may never come around. Your call is to just present the information. It's their choice whether to use it or not.

Just remember that as you continue to cultivate and tend your life-soil, no matter what bad seeds show up, you can still grow and thrive, and produce the best, most amazing life-fruit possible. Trust me, amazing fruit will grow, and when it does, it will be a glorious, prosperous and bountiful harvest. Keep in mind that you will always reap what you sow, so the more work and effort you put into it, the more you'll get in the end.

Ok, now that we know what we have to do, let's get to it! Let's start working on our perspective so that we can change our lives. Let's change our seat, and here's how!!

ACTION PLAN:

1. Be Honest: When creating your Roadmap to Wellness plan, you have to be honest with yourself in order to know where you are and where you want to be. Be careful though, do not be mean or belittle yourself: just be honest. If you step on the scale and find that you are 275 lbs., the reality is that you are 275 lbs. Accept it; and move forward.

    a. Don't overwhelm yourself thinking about all the things that you are doing wrong. In other words, let go of stinkin' thinkin'. Every time you have a negative thought about some aspect of your health, write it down. Just beneath it or next to it, write a positive statement about that thing.

        i. Example: "Diabetes runs in my family, so I was bound to get it" can be changed to, "Many people in my family have been diagnosed with diabetes, but we can, and will, change. We are winners!!"

2. How do you want the world to be different because you live in it? You are already a beautiful, wonderful gift to the world just by your mere presence. So, what kind of legacy do you want to leave?   Are you supposed to rebuild a community, start an international campaign to fight hunger, open a community center to help teach the children in the neighborhood to learn to read, or raise your own family to become a political powerhouse? Maybe you don't know yet, but the more you explore and ask this question, the more evident it will become and the more likely you will be able to step into your power.

3. Create a vision board: A vision board, simply put, is a visual representation of goals that you want to achieve in your life. The thought is that, by seeing your goals on a regular basis you will concentrate your time and energy on them and become less distracted from your daily grind. Vision boards are thought to help 1) identify your vision and give it clarity, 2) reinforce your daily affirmations, and 3) keep your attention on your intentions. This concept is not new by any means. You've heard phrases like "Keep your eyes on the prize" and "Ask and it shall be given, seek and you will find." All have the same underlying meaning: if you want it, you have to focus on it and go for it. Of course, this vision board project can go much more in depth and detail than I am presenting here.   Vision boards can actually be quite elaborate; however, don't try to be too elaborate at first. Vision boards are merely a starting point to get you moving in the direction of your goals.

Ok, so here are a few tips to get you started:

a. Choose your medium: You can create a vision board with almost anything from cardboard, construction paper, and butcher paper to bulletin boards. These, once completed, can be put on the wall of your office, bedroom, etc. You can also find websites that will help you build boards that you can look at on your computer. You can even purchase software that will allow you to do this. Decide where you most want to put your board. Remember that you can have more than one (it's even encouraged so that you will have better focus on each goal).

b. Find pictures of things you want to have or want to achieve. Don't just get the typical pictures (big house, fancy car, wad of cash, slim body, beautiful man/woman, etc.); find pictures that actually speak to you. Thumb through magazines or websites and notice those photos that make your heart race, hold your attention, or cause a double take. These are the images that should surround you. You can also find pictures of inspirational people whose footsteps you'd like to follow in some way. I once had pictures of Oprah and Maya Angelou on my board because they are powerful, intelligent women who are extremely successful in their respective areas.

c. Find words that inspire you. Cut out the words, and add them to your board. While I was in school, on one of my vision boards, I had words like "Top Doc" and "The Doctor Will See You Now" to help motivate me through school because completing school was my goal.

d. Choose your categories: What areas do you want to work on? I know; I know… "Everything!" But remember vision boards are used to create focus. Write down the categories that you want to focus on, then, if need be, rank them in order in which you want to start working on first, second, and so on. Categories can include

   i. Finances: Don't limit your financial success with the thought that having money will make you a bad, selfish, and/or evil person. Money only intensifies who you are, so if you are a giving person, think of how much more you can give and do if you just had the financial resources to do so!! Focus on the ways you can create more wealth, what it will take to maintain it, and the ways you can help others.

ii.   Relationships: Include all relationships, not just what you want the woman or man on your arm to look like. Include relationships with your children (current or future), extended family, co-workers, and friends. You can even include yourself. What type of relationship do you want to have with you? Are you the best you to you that you want you to be??

iii. Mental-Emotional Health: On www.HowToMakeAVisionBoard.com emotional health is discussed. One article on the site mentioned the following, *"Emotions can often determine whether we act out of inspiration or desperation. If fear and doubt are controlling your decisions, and thereby controlling your life direction, create a vision board that will serve as a constant reminder of who you are -- not where you have been but where you intend to be."*

iv.   Physical Health: Is there an activity that you used to do and want to start again? Is there a sport or activity you want to learn? Then just do it. Learn to eat, cook and enjoy different foods. Start your own garden to have more fresh produce available to you. Laugh and play more. Yes, really. All of the aforementioned can be added to the physical health section of your vision board.

v.   Spiritual: What were you put on earth to do? Are you fulfilling your purpose? Is there a spiritual disconnect between you and your higher power? Find ways to strengthen your spiritual health in order to help you fulfill your purpose. If you don't know your purpose, think about all the things that you want to do or that you feel drawn to do. Eventually, you will discover your ultimate purpose.

e. Remember that you don't have to have your entire life's goals planned out in detail when you create your board. Just have the main goals, stay focused, and move forward. Most important, have FUN creating the person that you want to see as you realize your goals!

4. Clear the Clutter: Lao Tzu, an ancient Chinese philosopher, once wrote, "To become learned, each day add something. To become enlightened, each day drop something." In response to that, Martha Beck, a writer for Oprah's OWN, wrote the following, "How much junk could a chic chick chuck if a chic chick could chuck junk?" In other words, if you want to learn more, do more, or be happier, then you've got to let some stuff go. If you want to have new things (ideas, mindsets, money, friends, etc.), you've got to get rid of some of the old things in order to make room for the new. Now, how do we get rid of the old to make way for the new? Glad you asked.

a. Start easy. Start with your car. It's a small space, but you probably spend a significant amount of time there. You can also get almost immediate benefit. Clean out the front of your car beginning with the driver's and passenger's seats. Then move to the glove compartment, dash and console. Next, you can move to the back seat and ash trays. Once that's done and when you're ready, tackle the trunk. Take your time and don't stress out. If your trunk is particularly cluttered, start with a bag, box or handful of items.

b. Desk: Organize your desk at work or home. Put things in stacks and piles so that you know roughly what's in each pile. Make the piles neat, but don't make them too large. Then, whenever you have a moment, go through each piece. Focus on one pile at a time if you can. File, trash, shred, sign, mail, and respond to each thing that is there. Again, don't overwhelm yourself. Just do what you can when you have a few spare minutes. Continue to do whatever it is that you need to do through the day. You'll find that you are getting through things much easier when they are organized and you are focusing on one task at a time, even in your spare time.

c. Do SPRING CLEANING!! Spring is the time for renewal, growth, and new beginnings. Spring cleaning is the time for getting rid of old things that weigh you and your home down and making room for the fresh new things that come into your home and your life. The great thing is that you can "spring clean" any time of year. There are many websites that can help you organize your cleaning project, but here is a brief overview. Pick a room and then section it off (Kitchen: drawers, cabinets, stove, and pantry). Bathroom: drawers, cabinet, counter. Bedroom: closets, drawers, under the bed, etc.) and focus on each section one-by-one. Then create four categories/boxes: Throw Away, Give away/Sell, Store, Keep. Every time you go through a part of your home, you will use these boxes to organize your things.

   i. Throw Away: things that you don't need or want and other people can't use. Include anything that is damaged or broken (no, you will NOT fix that later!! It's already been in there for 7 years. It's time for it to go! It's not worth keeping. Chuck it!)

   ii. Give away/Sell: These are things that you don't want but are in good repair so someone else may get some good use out of it. If you want to organize a garage sale, you can make some money off those newfound treasures. If you don't, you can just give those items to your local charity and receive a tax write off for your cleaning efforts. You can help others while you are helping yourself.

    iii. Store: Put away those things that you cannot part with but don't use on a regular basis. Try not to put everything in this category, though. Simply use it for those things that are out of season (clothing, shoes, comforters, etc.) or heirlooms. Label each box with the items in it so that you can easily retrieve them when you need to.

    iv. Keep: this should be your smallest category. These are items that you use on a regular basis. Make sure that you are not re-cluttering the area that these things come from. If the space becomes cluttered, try to reassess each item to ensure that you really need it, otherwise put it in one of the other categories.

  d. Working one area at a time makes it easier to come to a stopping point when necessary. When you come to a stopping point, immediately throw out the trash, put away the storage items, place the giveaway/sell items out of site or bring them to the donation facility. By doing this right away, you don't have an opportunity to reconsider anything and possibly put it back where you got it from.

  e. Once an area is de-cluttered, make a conscious effort not to put anything in it that doesn't belong. Keeping the space clear on a regular basis makes it much easier to maintain.

5. Affirm it!! Self-Affirmations, according to WikiHow.com, are "positive statements or self-scripts that can condition the subconscious mind so that you can develop a more positive perception of yourself." Affirmations are positive statements or

judgments. They can help you change your thinking by replacing negative thoughts and self-perceptions into positive ones. They are mantras that you can repeat on a regular basis. By repeating these statements, you are creating beliefs that your conscious and subconscious selves will eventually begin to hold on to and use in every aspect of your life. Self-affirmations help to build self-esteem, and they help keep you focused on your goals without getting discouraged. There are several ways that affirmations can be used. You can both find and use some that were created by others, you can create ones that you believe will impact you, or you can find your own negative self-talk and reword it to become positive self-talk.

   a. Here are a few Affirmations that I ran across and I thought were powerful statements. If they resonate with you, say them often, especially in times where your positivity is less than perfect.

      i. I am too big a gift to this world to feel self-pity and sadness.

      ii. I am uniquely beautiful.

      iii. I have a healthy spirit, mind, and body.

      iv. I am full of energy and vitality.

      v. My mind is calm and peaceful.

      vi. I am free of unwanted stress.

      vii. My body heals quickly and easily.

      viii. I love learning about and experimenting with new foods.

      ix. God's light and love flows through every cell of my body.

   b. Here's a simple way to create your own affirmations and mantras:

      i. Think of your positive attributes: Take a look at all the wonderful things you like about yourself or that others have complimented you on. Do you like your smile? Do you have beautiful eyes? Are you giving to others? By focusing on the good things, you can begin to break the cycle of focusing solely on the negative things about yourself. Begin to write these down in simple statements beginning each with "I" and put them in the present tense. For example, "I have a radiant smile" or "I have beautiful eyes" or "I am a generous person."

ii.   Think about the negative things you tell yourself repeatedly and the things you would like to change. List each of these on a sheet of paper and prioritize them. Example: lose weight, quite smoking, improve self-confidence, etc. You can work on as many of these as you want, but again you don't want to overwhelm yourself. Try not to focus on more than 3-5 at a time. These can be in line with your overall *ROADMAP TO SUCCESS* plans. Now let's rewrite them.

iii. Writing the Affirmations: Now that you've had practice writing your positive qualities, you can use this same format to create the 'counter scripts' in order to counteract the negative thoughts. The affirmations you create will all be in the present tense and begin with the word "I". They fall into two basic categories: 'I can' and 'I will'.

   1. "I can" statements bring to reality all the things that you can do. When creating these, avoid using any negative terms like "not," for example: 'I can stop smoking," or "I can become smoke-free."

   2. "I will" statements are more like action statements that you will focus on that day. Again, avoid using negative terms

when creating these. "I will smoke fewer cigarettes today than yesterday" is a good statement. You want to avoid saying, "I will *not* smoke as many cigarettes today." Saying, "I will eat 3 servings of leafy green veggies today" is a better option than "I will *not* eat processed foods today."

iv. Make your affirmations visible: Put your statements somewhere that you will see them regularly. Write them on sticky notes and post them in obvious places in your home, car and workspace. Carry them in your purse or wallet so that you can read them when you need a pick-me-up.

v. Use them daily: Take a few moments several times a day to meditate and focus on these positive statements. Write affirmations in a journal as soon as you wake up and just before you go to bed. Write and use them often to help solidify them in your mind and consciousness.

"There is nothing like returning to a place that remains unchanged to find the ways in which you yourself have altered" - Nelson Mandela

CHAPTER 4

What's So Funny?

Cʒ ৪০

A Joyful heart is good medicine, but a crushed spirit dries up the bones. ~Proverbs 17:22

Stop being so serious all the time!! Life is too short to take yourself so seriously every moment of every day. It's time to learn to lighten up. Live a little. Laugh a lot! You deserve it.

Laughter is your birthright! Babies begin smiling within weeks, and sometimes even days, of being born. People often say "That's just gas", but isn't that the happiest, most wonderful gas you ever saw? Shouldn't we all be so happy when we fart?

It's been found that little children giggle an average of 400 times a day. Unfortunately, as we get older, as we go through life, we grow out of that wonderful habit. Adults on average only laugh about 15 times a day. It's really important that we all get back into the habit of enjoying our lives **on purpose**. We need to start to do more laughing, smiling and giggling and less frowning and scowling.

Have you ever gotten so angry with someone, I mean really, *REALLY* angry with someone, that you couldn't even look in their general direction without wanting to punch them in the left shoulder? Didn't you want to be angry all day? Don't you just hate it when that same person says or does something to make you smile? Once you smile, that's it. You can no longer hold that grudge against them. Things lighten up, even if only a little bit and for just a short period of time, they lighten up. That's the beauty of laughing and smiling. It releases all that stress, anxiety and anger that is building up and causing so many problems internally. It lightens your burden. It gives you hope and keeps you focused.

Laughter is the best medicine – unless you're diabetic, then insulin comes pretty high on the list -Jasper Carrott

Laughter really is good medicine. Research has shown that there are actually a myriad of health benefits that laughter provides. Don't believe me? Well, check out this list of all the things laughter does:

- ✓ Massages your internal organs
- ✓ Strengthens your abdominal muscles
  - o *Hearty laughter is a good way to jog internally without having to go outdoors ~Norman Cousins*
- ✓ Releases stress for up to 45 minutes, thereby protecting you from the harmful effects of stress
- ✓ Releases serotonin, the 'feel good' hormone
- ✓ Protects the heart by improving blood vessel function and increasing blood flow
- ✓ Boosts the immune system
- ✓ Increases energy
- ✓ Relaxes muscles, which also helps improve blood flow
- ✓ Improves memory, creativity and alertness
- ✓ Increases oxygen intake
- ✓ Stimulates the heart and lungs
- ✓ Decreases pain
- ✓ Balances blood pressure
- ✓ Promotes relaxation
- ✓ Improves sleep
- ✓ May prevent and/or help heal cancer and other chronic illnesses
- ✓ Improves quality of life for those with chronic illnesses

- ✓ Diffuses conflict which can lengthen life (especially if someone was really, really angry!!)
- ✓ Releases endorphins, the body's endogenous painkillers
- ✓ Shifts your perspective
- ✓ Attracts others to you
- ✓ Provides a sense of overall well-being
- ✓ Is FREE!!

With a list like that, what's not to laugh about??

ACTION PLAN:

> *It is impossible for you to be angry and laugh at the same time. Anger and laughter are mutually exclusive and you have the power to choose either* ~ *Wayne Dyer*

It's unfortunate that we have to make a conscious effort to include more laughter in our lives, but it is a beautiful thing to realize that we need more laughter and are actually making that effort. Here are some ways to increase the amount of laughing that you do throughout your day and subsequently increase your overall health.

1. Smile: It's the first part of a laugh, right? If need be, give yourself reminders to smile. Smile as often as possible. Smiling is contagious, so spread it around. Remember, it's better to develop smile lines than frown lines.

2. Learn a new joke: Make it a really corny one! Tell it as often as you can, and watch the reactions you get. Think about it, how funny is it when someone gives you that blank, confused stare when they are trying not to hurt your feelings? Consider this, the joke you are telling is primarily for your benefit, not theirs. So, the joke's on them.

3. Host a Game Night with your friends: Go to the thrift store and purchase a bunch of your favorite games. Make it a mix of childhood games and adult games. Invite a few fun friends over and just play for hours. Trust me; going from *Pictionary* to

Candy Land to *Spades* to *Sorry* is a whirlwind of good times and laughs.

4. Go sing karaoke in front of strangers: Pick your favorite song, even if you don't know the words, get on stage, and sing loudly. Just sing. Perform. Give them a show. You may not even look at the words. Just sing the wrong words. Who cares? Enjoy yourself.

5. Go roller skating, and laugh when you fall on your butt. As a friend of mine once told her daughter, "Falling is half the fun of skating."

6. Find Laughter regularly: make an effort to do something that will take your mind off things and make you laugh in the meantime.

   a. Watch an old movie
   b. Read a comic book
   c. Cuddle with kittens – or puppies if you have allergies – or salamanders if you don't like either of those – or cacti if you just really don't like animals.
   d. Watch an entire season of your favorite sitcom
   e. Play with little children. Since they laugh all the time, you may be infected with their joy and laughter multiple times. Call it 'joy-gasms'. LOL!!!!!! That made me laugh.
   f. Go to a comedy show: There are great local comedians that are extremely funny in many of these comedy clubs. Go out and laugh at these unknown comedians. Who knows, maybe you'll meet a new friend and have regular laughs together. If there's no comedy club in your area, try Comedy Central. It's 24 hour laughter at your fingertips.

7. Laugh Yoga: Yes, there are actually classes out there where people get together and laugh intentionally. Leave all your cares and hang-ups behind and join a group of people that also know that laughter is good medicine.

8. Put things in proper perspective: Are situations in your life really **that** serious? Do you really need to frown all the time? Is that really your problem or does it actually belong to someone else? Will it kill you to lighten up a bit? Even the Grinch, with his tiny, hardened heart, didn't die when his heart started to grow, and he started to smile more. I'm pretty sure that you won't either.

9. Find a Happy Crew: Surround yourself with people that truly enjoy life. They don't have to be your close friends (besides, if your close friends did more fun, happy stuff you probably wouldn't have to try to find more laughter, right?). Find people that have good, clean fun, play games, and are not so ridged. Remember the saying, "Birds of a feather flock together?" If you surround yourself with light hearted, fun, happy birds you will become more like them and begin to find yourself smiling more.

10. YouTube it: Go on YouTube and type in "Laughing Babies" or "Cute Kittens" or "Playful Puppies." Take a few moments and appreciate the innocence and simplicity of those young ones.

11. Make it a Blockbuster Night: Get together with a friend or two and rent a movie. Rent one that none of you have seen before. Go to the house and watch the movie. Here's the twist: you should watch the movie in silence. Just mute the entire movie. Then, each of you pick a character or two or three and create your own dialogue, complete with different voices and all.

12. Call a childhood friend and remind him or her about a song or phrase or event that used to keep you in stitches. Better yet, send your friend a random text message or email with a phrase, music lyrics, or word that used to make you laugh. Trust me when I say it's a great joy to read those unexpected messages, but it's also fun sending them!

The bottom line is that it's time to find more joy. It doesn't have to be complicated. It's as important to have joy and laughter as it is to drink water and breathe. Know that *"Nobody ever died of laughter" (Max*

Beerbohm) but lots of folks could have lived longer, healthier, happier lives if they would have made an effort to laugh more.

It's up to you to create, or re-create, the happiness that you want and deserve. Remember, joy and happiness are your birthright. If you've given up that birthright somewhere along the way, then it's time to reclaim it!!

So, in the immortal words of that great poet and singer, Bobby McFerrin, "Don't Worry, Be Happy".

You can turn painful situations around through laughter. If you can find humor in anything, even poverty, you can survive it. ~ Bill Cosby

CHAPTER 5

Empty Your Trash!

❦ ❧

"Happiness is found in pooping, not merely possessing."
– (adapted from) Napoleon Hill

Have you ever looked at someone and thought, "You are so full of $*@%!!" Well... if it was a typical American eating a Standard American Diet (SAD), you were probably right. Most people that you see are clogged up, having less than 1 bowel movement per day and sometimes only a few a week, IF that many.

I've heard many people say, "... but that's *my* normal." I must admit that I've even been guilty of saying it myself, before I knew better. Having infrequent bowel movements may be your normal, but that is by no means what should be occurring in your body for optimal health. On top of that, your normal may actually be helping to decrease your level of health.

Those of us that study and practice Naturopathic Medicine, "Complimentary and Alternative Medicine", and natural healing know that health and disease begins in the digestive system. The better you are at breaking down foods, absorbing nutrients and getting rid of waste products, the better your overall health will be. The better you breakdown, absorb and assimilate those nutrients the more resources your body has available for proper function. The more efficient you are at removing and eliminating waste from your cells, tissues, and organs the more space and energy your body has to do what it needs to do in order to make and keep you well.

Think about it this way. What happens if you leave your dinner, let's say steak and potatoes with rice and gravy, on your linoleum floors at a temperature around 100 degrees (close to body temperature) for days and weeks at a time? Well for starters it will start to stink pretty quickly. It will get infested with bugs and bacteria and eventually mold. I'm pretty sure that it will also start to ruin your linoleum as well. The floor beneath the food will start to become discolored; the waxy coat will start to erode, and the food will eventually start to eat/burn its way through the tile causing holes. That's not a very pleasant thought is it? Now think about this. How much more delicate is your body than that floor?

Did you know that over half of your immune system as well as your feel good hormones are produced and used in the area of your digestive system? If the GI (Gastrointestinal / Digestive) system is off and not working properly, most likely your immune functions and your happy hormone production are not functioning properly either.

Other correlations to consider are these:

- When your colon is full, your body tends to feel heavier, because you are carrying dead weight …literally. You can become more lethargic and less comfortable. The worst part of having a full colon is that many people don't even realize just how heavy and lethargic they feel because they are always so full.
- There is a very strong correlation between health of your GI system and the appearance of your skin. The more constipated a person is, the more likely he or she is to experience problems like acne, dull, dry skin, pimples, etc. If the colon and other organs of elimination (kidneys, lungs, liver, etc.) are back logged, the body will have to recycle wastes until it can get rid of them in any way that it can. This backlog can manifest itself as skin issues because the skin is the largest organ of elimination that humans have.

- Bad breath: if a person's breath smells like a toilet, most likely they need to go to the toilet!
- If you are overweight, then you are 'over waste'. Many of the trash, metabolites and toxins that are inside our body are fat soluble. If your body doesn't know what to do with them or doesn't have the capacity to get rid of it soon, then those things can be stored in the fat tissue. By making it easier and more efficient for things to exit the body, you make it easier to get rid of any byproducts - like the waste products created from everyday activities of the cells, old hormones, environmental pollutants, etc. If you get rid of them, the body doesn't have to try to store this material allowing you to lose weight with much more ease.

Optimally, every time you eat something you should go to the bathroom a short time later. Even if you are not eliminating quite that often, one good movement a day without straining will suffice, as long as it is about equal to the amount of food you ate the day before. What exits your body should be about equivalent to what enters your body. If you are eating quarter pound burgers and not getting rid of a quarter pound of waste, what do you think happens to it? Don't be a big eater and a small pooper!

> *"In my world everyone is a pony, and they all eat rainbows, and poop butterflies."* ~ Horton Hears a Who!

ACTION PLAN:

Of course, there are several approaches that can help you begin to eliminate more completely, many more than are being provided in this chapter. If you and your spouse are not getting the results you want, contact your Naturopathic Physician or other health care provider for more individualized support.

1. Drink water! Often times we are just dry. Drink more water and herbal teas so that more water is available for proper elimination. Try to avoid those beverages that have a lot of ingredients, sugars, and other additives in them. The more additives and sugars, the more likely they are to dehydrate you than hydrate. Check out Chapter 9 for ways to increase your water/fluid intake.

2. Probiotics, the "Good Bacteria": These little buggers are the cornerstone of good health within your body and within your colon! They help improve your digestion, they produce some of the vitamins that you cannot produce on your own, and they help to regulate and boost your immune system. Many people suffer from constipation or diarrhea, especially if they've ever taken antibiotics (which kill both bad and good bacteria), because they don't have an adequate amount of beneficial bacteria in their system. You can repopulate your system with these helpful little guys simply and easily. You will be amazed at how efficiently you digest your food and how your health reacts when you have all the right workers on the inside!

    a. Eat yogurt that contains "live cultures" in it. Try to stay away from those that already have fruit and syrup in them. Purchase plain yogurt (like Greek yogurt) and add your own fruit, granola, nuts, and natural sweeteners like raw honey, pure maple syrup, or stevia. I've found that the plain yogurts tend to be less expensive and allow you to be more creative. You also know exactly what is going into your body! Kefir is a similar product you might also try.

    b. Eat fermented, unpasteurized foods: Traditional foods like sauerkraut, kimchee, pickled veggies, and real root beer are just a few examples of how you can include fermented unpasteurized foods in your diet. You can even try making some of the foods yourself. Check Chapter 13 for a few recipes.

3. Increase fiber: Fiber is like the broom that sweeps and cleans out your insides. The typical Western diet contains very little soluble or insoluble fiber. Most people will get only about 15 grams of fiber, if they are lucky. Since this is the case, you may have to make a special effort to get more fiber into your body. The optimal range of fiber intake is 25-35 grams per day. This may sound like a lot, but if you break it down and modify your dietary intake, it doesn't have to be difficult. Here are some healthy and easy ways to get fiber in

    a. 1 cup oatmeal is 4 g fiber
    b. ½ banana is 1.5g
    c. 1 tbsp. flax seeds (whole or freshly ground) is 2.8 g
    d. Snacking on 25 Almonds (~3.5g) + ¼ cup Raisins (~1.5g) will easily give you 5g of fiber
    e. Greek yogurt, with all of its 'good bacteria' and ½ cup blueberries gives you 2 g of fiber and a very happy tummy.
    f. 1 small apple has 4.4g
    g. 3 cups of popcorn (skip the excess butter and salt and sugar) is easily 3.5 g
    h. ½ cup lentils can give you 10g - 20g fiber
    i. ½ cup black beans is 10g fiber
    j. 1 cup brown rice is 3.5 grams
    k. ½ cup Quinoa is 5g fiber.
    l. 1 tbsp. Ch-ch-ch-CHIA Seeds packs 10g of fiber. You can add them to your lemonade (for Chia Fresca) or your yogurt, oatmeal or cereal for an extra boost of fiber
    m. 1 cup shredded romaine lettuce is 1g
    n. 1 cup spinach is 0.7g
    o. ½ cup grated carrots has 1.6g
    p. ¼ cup walnuts has 4g
        i. Putting it together:
            1. Breakfast: 1 cup oatmeal + ½ banana + 1 tbsp. flax seeds = 8.5g Fiber

2. Midday Snack: 25 almonds + ¼ cup raisins = 5g fiber
3. Lunch: Medium salad with 1 cup Romaine, 1 cup Spinach, ½ cup grated carrots, and ¼ cup walnuts = 7g.
   Lunch: ½ cup lentils + ½ cup brown rice = about 15g
4. Evening Snack: 3 cups plain popcorn = 3.5g
5. Dinner: 1 cup black beans + 1 cup quinoa = 20g
   Dessert: 1 cup Greek yogurt + ½ cup blueberries + 1 tbsp. Chia seeds = 12g
6. Added total Fiber for that day you'll get 71 grams of fiber!!!!!! How simple was that??

4. Move Something! The more your outsides move, the more your insides move. Walking, running, playing, and deep breathing all cause an increase in smooth muscle contractions not only of your legs, but also of your core (abs). The organs underneath can benefit because they get a massage every time your muscles move. The tightening and relaxing of the muscles helps to reinforce and encourage the muscular function of the intestines and other organs which leads to better waste elimination.

5. Get in the SQUAT Position: There are devices called "squat stools" that are designed to be put in front of your toilet so that you can prop your feet up in a position that simulates a squat (the position that we used to get into to release our waste, before the advent of modern toilets). When we get into the squat position, the muscles of our pelvis and lower part of our colon change position such that it becomes easier for the body to release waste [FYI: this is also the natural position women get into in order to give birth with more ease]. If you don't want to invest in a squatting stool, you can simply purchase a step stool

from any local store (I got mine from a dollar store). You can also just stack phone books (if they still make them??), prop your foot up on an overturned trash can, or on the side of the tub. The whole point is to elevate your feet so that your knees are somewhat above your pelvis. I have friends that thought I was nuts when I first told them about it, but now they swear by it!!

    a. Interesting Fact: I just found out that if a person has a spinal cord injury and they don't have bowel function, this is the recommended position to increase peristalsis – the wavelike movement of the intestines that helps move the waste out. (Thanks Lisa!!)

6. Relax and Breathe: When I first read about the squatting position for elimination and I read we should relax, breathe, and "feel the peace of your release," it sounded kind of 'woo woo' at the time. But I did what the author suggested, and guess what? As crazy as it sounded, the author was right. There was no straining, no effort, just a peaceful release. Just the way it should be! Next time you need to go, make an effort *not* to strain. Take a relaxing inhale for the count of 4 and exhale for the count of 8. While you are exhaling, release all the tension, negativity, poop and all the other things you want to get rid of. You'll find that it begins to take less effort to eliminate, and you'll also avoid hemorrhoids in the process. Check out Chapter 6 for more breathing techniques that you can use throughout your day to help you relax.

CHAPTER 6

Just Breathe

C8 80

To control the breathing is to control the mind. With different patterns of breathing, you can fall in love, you can hate someone, and you can feel the whole spectrum of feelings just by changing your breathing. — Marina Abramovic

You may be asking yourself why I have a section that focuses on breathing. I mean, we all breathe all the time, right? Because if we didn't breathe we wouldn't be alive, right? If you are asking these questions then you are absolutely correct, AND, you are also absolutely incorrect. Let me explain.

When you breathe, are you really taking breaths, or are you just slowly panting? Are you taking full, deep breaths? Are you using ALL of your lung space to take in fresh air and get rid of the stale, used up air? Did you just take a deep breath as you were reading that last sentence? If the answer is yes, then most likely, you aren't breathing properly.

Breathing, taking in those nice, slow, deep breaths, is hugely beneficial. Generally, the more stressed out and hectic our lives get the more shallow and quick our inhalations become. When this happens, you are depriving your blood of oxygen. That in and of itself can cause stress to the body because your cells are now trying to work in less-than-optimal conditions. Now, because your cells are more stressed, you begin to breathe more shallowly, which leads to less oxygen, which leads to…. a vicious cycle of high stress and low oxygen. After a while, it becomes hard to tell where the cycle began. At some point, it really doesn't matter. What matters is that you stop the cycle, even if for only a few moments a day in the beginning.

At one of the local colleges, I taught a course in Exercise Biochemistry. Basically, the class went over many of the processes that occur at a cellular and sub-cellular level as it relates to exercise. Important points we discussed were the importance of activity and how movement affects the different chemicals – hormones, enzymes, vitamins, minerals, etc – in the body.

There is one process that the body goes through called "Oxidative Phosphorylation." This is a process that occurs deep inside the cells. This chemical reaction is how your cells produce ATP, the main energy currency needed for the cell to function. Basically, in this reaction, the body uses oxygen to create the energy that is needed. It's during this process that our cells make the highest volume of ATP currency.

Why is that important? Well, if a body does not have adequate oxygen, then it cannot create the maximum amount of energy. The less air and oxygen that are taken in, the more 'anaerobic' the body can become and the less energy will be made. Our bodies don't function best in these conditions. Being anaerobic can lead to decreased performance, low endurance, and a high amount of fatigue. This (production of large amounts of energy) is why we breathe!

Lack of oxygen also causes a decrease in blood flow throughout tissues. This decrease in blood flow causes muscles to tense up which leads to less blood flow. Vicious cycle, anyone?

After a while, shallow breathing becomes a bad habit that can be really hard to break. So we should treat it like any other bad habit, start slow and build.

One way to break up any kind of tension is good deep breathing –
Byron Nelson

ACTION PLAN:

Here are some ways to modify your breathing to help improve your health and wellbeing.

- Set the timer on your phone for 3-5 minutes. Sit in a chair with both feet on the floor. Put your hands on your lap. Close your eyes. Block out everything around you and everything going on in your head. Take a slow, deep inhale for the count of four (remember to count slowly! "1-2-3-4"), then exhale slowly, in a relaxed manner for the count of four, "4-3-2-1". Repeat this slow breathing for the duration of time, until the alarm goes off. Pick a time of day that this breathing exercise will be most beneficial and consistent for you, like when you wake up, before bed, or at your desk at work.

- As you get used to this breathing exercise the length of time will get easier for you and allow you to increase the breathing timeframe by 30-60 seconds. Example: if you are breathing for 3 minutes, and you found it particularly challenging, then after the exercise 5-6 times a week for several weeks, add 30 seconds. Then after a few weeks add 30 more seconds. If you did 5 minutes with ease, 5-7 times a week then increase your breathing time by 60 seconds.

- Add a second time to do your breathing exercises, choosing times that will benefit you most – waking and before bed; when you first get to work and when you first get home after work; when you first get home from work and just before bed, etc. Do what is most convenient and beneficial for you.

- Once you get comfortable with the breathing exercises, you can start using the technique at any time during the day that you feel particularly stressed. Try your focused breathing while you are in traffic (with your eyes open of course!), sitting at your computer screen, while cooking dinner, while paying bills, or even sitting in meetings.

- Increase the length of your exhalation from a four count to a 6 count. Eventually, lengthen your exhalation to an eight count.
- Increase the length of your inhalation from a four count to a 6 count. Then eventually increase it to an 8 count.
- Find some relaxing sounds or music to practice your breathing exercises. There are great nature sound CDs and videos that can be very useful. If you like ocean waves, rain drops, forest or other sounds like that, you'll do well investing in this to help you relax. You can also use drums, flutes, or some other music. Whatever it is that you resonate with, use that. It's preferable that you begin with music that has no words so that your attention can remain on your breath and not the words in the song.
- Pick up meditation CDs, find relaxation videos on YouTube, or search for breathing and relaxation apps on your smart phone. All these can be easily found and very useful in helping you focus on improving your relaxation techniques, as they guide you through the process. Check out Chapter 15 for a few Smartphone apps that I've found to be pretty helpful.

Remember that these changes don't all need to be done at the same time. After you've mastered (or at least gotten used to) one of them, pick a variation and work it into your routine until it becomes more comfortable for you. Then add another. You'll be amazed at how great a simple change like breathing can help every aspect of your life.

> *I wake up every day and I think, 'I'm breathing! It's a good day.'* -Eve Ensler

CHAPTER 7

You've Got to Move It, Move It

CB EO

Walking is man's best medicine – Hippocrates

Motion is one of the most fundamental parts of life. Motion *is* life.   In order for anything on Earth to be alive, there must be motion, either internal or external or some combination of them both.

When plants and beings are newly "born," they are in their most active time and are usually in the period of their most motion and growth. They are most supple. That is the case with everything from tree seedlings to infants to baby animals. It is when that being is closer to death that it starts to get hard, stiff, stagnant and rigid. In death, all motion ceases.

You can even see this play out with bodies of water. Those bodies of water that have a steady flow and are constantly being fed by tributaries have the most life. There are trees that flourish nearby as well, and grass and flowers are vibrant. Different types of aquatic life thrive within it. There are even animals and insects that come to visit in order to drink and bathe. It's a very lively, energetic place. Now, compare that to a puddle or some man-made lake that doesn't have a constant in and out flow of water. There may be some tadpoles. There may be an occasional bird that comes to drink and bathe, but for the most part, especially in comparison to the moving body of water, that one is stagnant. Over time, lack of motion results in rot and decay. The water will begin to smell putrid. There will be no vibrant colors surrounding it, and you'll probably have an infestation of bugs and mold. In other words, because there would be no life, everything would be dead.

And so it goes within your body. When you are born, you are full of energy. You play. You run. You move…. A LOT. As you get older, you slow down, and with society and technology at the level it is currently, you will sit for hours and hours at a time. Couple this with poor dietary choices, decreased oxygen intake and constipation (stagnation in the colon), and you've created a recipe for poor health.

The good news is that if this is the direction that you've been going, you CAN change course! You don't have to stay stagnant and dormant. You don't have to get stiff and slow down.

"Motion is Lotion"

One of my Physical Medicine instructors used to always say that motion was lotion. He always talked about how movement was needed to help heal stiff and ailing joints. In my experience, personal and professional, I've found that this is largely true. Motion *is* lotion. It may seem to be counterintuitive for some, but the very thing that is needed to help restore many of today's top ailments is increased movement. I was recently watching "The Doctors" on TV and Dr. Francis said, "The single best thing anyone can do when diagnosed with a problem is to exercise."

"You can't out exercise a bad diet" – FB Meme

If you happen to be dealing with some health malady that has been caused by, contributed to, or exacerbated by the lack of exercise you always want to remember that exercise and motion are just one part of the equation. Even if you are relatively healthy and you have other fitness, health or cosmetic goals to achieve, you should know that exercise alone won't get you nearly as far. The amount of calories you burn and the elevation of heart rate also represent an important component of your Roadmap to Success. Equally important is the fuel that you put into your body.

If you habitually put large amounts of poor quality foods that contain high amounts of calories from highly processed grains, concentrated sugars and low quality oils with little to no nutrient value, you won't see nearly the level of results that you want to see. You won't be able to experience the amounts of healing and rejuvenation that you could see if you were fueling your body with high quality foods that have appropriate caloric values and multiple nutrients that work synergistically with one another. In other words, a Twinkie, chips and a soda (even if it's diet…. ESPECIALLY if it's diet!) are still a Twinkie, chips and soda no matter how much time you spend in the gym. You may not see the effects of it as soon or as overtly if you exercise, but it will still affect you none-the-less. Be sure to check out Chapter 12 *"You Are What You Eat"* and Chapter 13, *"Let's Eat!"* for more information on why nutrition is important and ways to incorporate better foods into your day.

In an effort to increase the amount of motion you engage in regularly, there are a few things to keep in mind:

> Exercise doesn't equal "Gym": There's no need to get a membership to the local fitness facility in order to get physically active. Of course, gyms can be wonderful places to assist you in reaching your goals, but they are not a necessity. If you don't have the time or money to go to the gym or you are not comfortable working out next to the lady in the spandex or the guy with the bulging muscles, you don't have to. You can still get fabulous results!

> Don't overcomplicate it: Start off simple and add to your baseline as you improve. You are much more likely to reach your goals with small, consistent steps than you are with big, weekend-warrior type exercising. Remember that slow and steady wins the race.

> Don't overthink it: This is one of my personal struggles. I often have great plans and wonderful ideas, but sometimes they will get delayed because I'm exhausted before I even get started.

Or I will add so many variables to what it is that I am trying to do that by the end, I need a support team and a large budget to even start the task. If that sounds even remotely like you, then we both need to STOP IT! Always remember the K.I.S.S. philosophy: Keep It Simple, Superstar!!

➤ Start where you are: You may not be able to get up and start training for the Boston Marathon right away. You may not even be able to get up right away. Both are ok. Focus on what you *can* do. I've found many chair exercise videos on TV, YouTube, and DVD that I've given to my less mobile patients. I've also found many yoga videos that are good for stretching and strengthening specific areas of the body that may be weaker. I even found a workout book (it happened to be on sale at a bookstore) that showed exercises that could be done with 1 Gallon jugs filled with differing amounts of water as weights. The point is that you are not destined to be sedentary just because you are now. You just need a bit of creativity and an equal amount of motivation.

➤ Consistency is key: Being consistent is much more important than going hard and heavy and fast. Again, slow and steady wins the race.

➤ Find someone to play with: Get support. Doing things alone isn't always the best option. Sometimes we need the support and encouragement of others to help push us through the tough times and praise us in the good times. You can get your family and coworkers to join you or find a group of strangers that have similar goals.

➤ Have some fun: You are much more likely to be enthusiastic and consistent about things you enjoy. So go out and find fun stuff to do. New things. Old things. Just have fun. It is so much easier when you are doing activities you enjoy.

➤ You have to make the effort: No matter how much I talk about how easy it is, no matter how many gadgets you purchase from the exciting infomercials, and no matter how many groups you join the bottom line is that nothing will change until you take the first step (then the second, third, fourth…..).

Ok. Now, let's get moving!! Let's figure out some ways to have you increase your mobility without overdoing it and while having fun at the same time!

ACTION PLAN:

1. The first thing to do is to write down how many times a week that you will *realistically* incorporate more movement. If you are a sedentary person (you sit for hours a day and the only movement you really get is to and from the car and from one room to the other), then start with a couple days a week for a few minutes each time. Of course, ideally you want to move 5-7 days a week for at least 30 minutes at a time, but the reality is that for many people that amount of time is physically and/or mentally impossible to start out with. So, that amount of time can be one of your goals, but it doesn't have to be where you start. If you are already very active, figure out ways that you can increase your activity. As you get healthier and more fit, begin to add 5-10 minutes to your workout time. Then add another day/time, and then increase your intensity. The more you do it, the easier it gets to incorporate into your life because it is a part of your life and not something that you are trying to fit in.

The rest of this section is dedicated to giving you ideas on more ways to incorporate activity. No matter what you do, remember the adage, "No pain. No gain" is only partially right. You want to work your body so that it can become stronger (this will give you a bit of muscle soreness) but if it outright hurts, then you are doing too much too soon. Back up and slow down until you get stronger.

2. Walk it out: The only requirement for walking is YOU. Get up. Get out. Go! When walking, try to do more than a leisurely

stroll around the neighborhood. Do enough to get your heart rate elevated. If you are an elder, have been immobile for a while, or are extremely sedentary then the leisurely stroll may be enough for now. Decide how long you will walk, or pick a certain distance to strive for and go. If you don't make your goal the first day, that's ok. Keep working on it and don't give up. As you continue, you will get better at walking around, and you will go longer and further. As you improve, consider adding 2-5 minutes to your walk time. If you have distance goals (instead of time goals) add a quarter mile at a time as you get stronger. To help you keep track of your time and distance goals, find a Smartphone app that records your time. There are even those that have GPS so that you can chart your course and log your distance.

3. Have more SEX: Ok, now of course I'm talking ONLY to those people that are in monogamous, loving (at least I hope it's loving), devoted relationships! Because, no one else would be even considering sex, right??? ☺ So, if you are in a relationship, one of the best ways to get more active and grow closer in your relationship is to increase your physical intimacy. Have sex more often and for longer periods of time. Be creative. Change it up. Fantasize. Role play. Spice things up. When you have sex, you are not only having sex, but you are also releasing many different hormones that can help you relax, release stress, relax and exercise your muscles, help the two of you bond, protect and strengthen your heart and other organs, etc. Again, the main two points are to increase your activity and have FUN!!!

4. Stretch: Stretching is imperative to increase blood flow to every area of your body. It keeps your muscles pliable and helps you stay young (especially since you will not be as stiff and stagnant). You can always do your basic stretches. You know the exercises you used to do in your school gym class? Yes, do those. Hold the stretch for a while so that your body can relax and sink into the stretch. Stretch as many of your large and

small muscles as you can. You can also try something like yoga and Pilates. There are various types of each with various levels of intensity. Make no mistake about it, yoga and Pilates can get you very strong, very stretched, and very healthy!!   And yoga and Pilates aren't just for the ladies. Even men who are athletes benefit greatly from these type exercises because it allows their bodies to stretch and workout in non-impact ways. It's a great way to cross train for any and every one. It also helps you with #3!! ☺

5. DANCE! Have you noticed that no one dances much anymore? Do you remember how much you enjoyed it when you did? One of the easiest ways to get your heart rate up and have some fun is to turn up some good music on the stereo, or your iPod, and dance.   Dance around your living room, kitchen, bedroom... just dance. If you are home alone, dance naked! It can be very liberating!!

6. Take a dance class: if you're not the type to just break out dancing to your favorite music, then try taking a dance class. Take up a form of dancing that you've always wanted to try. Pick up a class that you used to take as a child. If you find that you don't like it, that's ok. Pick another one. You never know until you try. You may meet some great people that are fun to dance with in the process. How cool would that be to have regular dance partners and get some exercise in the process

7. Ride a bike: Riding a bike is like... well... riding a bike. If you haven't done it for a while, just get on and go. It'll all come back to you. Find a place that you can ride that will allow you to go a little faster. Go farther than you expected to go. Change the gear settings so that you increase the resistance. Enjoy your surroundings. Feel the breeze. Discover a new park. Ride through the forest. Riding can be an amazing way to burn calories, get active, see different parts of your neighborhood, and get some much needed alone time.

   ✓ An option is to get a tandem bike and ride with your partner. That can be an amazing bonding experience with someone you love while you both get in better shape!

✓ Another great option is to go to a cycling class at your local fitness facility. These workouts can be fantastic!!

8. Play with the children: Play with little ones (if they are not yours, ask the parents first, of course!). Really play with them, not as an adult, but as a human playing with a little human. Try to see the world from their point of view. Enjoy the little things. Discover. Run around. Use your imagination. Cultivate their imagination. Climb some trees. Play Tag, Red-light-Green-light, or Duck-duck-goose. Find and reconnect with your inner child by playing with children. It's very liberating to let your adult-self take a break from 'real world' issues and just have good, innocent fun for a while.

9. Play with adults: Have you noticed that adults don't play anymore? It's really unfortunate, but as we get older we tend to lose our fun side, or our fun becomes much more regulated and technological. It's time that we get out and get physical. Let go of your rigid ideas of what adults should and shouldn't do, and just have fun. Join a biking group, a jogging group, or a gardening group. Find a beginners racquetball league or take a swim class. Find a group of friends to play basketball, soccer, or touch football with. Maybe you can join a hiking group or a climbing club. Just go play!

10. Try something old: look into some of those activities that you did in your youth. You wouldn't believe how much energy it takes and how much health it can create! And it won't cost you much. Some examples of things you can do for some serious workouts are:

✓ Jump rope: You can burn 95 calories in 10 minutes! Remember that boxers use jumping rope to get that fancy footwork. It is a great cardio workout, it doesn't cost much, and you can take it anywhere!

✓ Hula hoop: The "Hula Hoop Man" (That's the name he goes by) in NYC Central park told me that you can get a six or 8 pack of abs if you just hula hooped every day for 30 minutes. You know why I believe him? Because he had an AMAZING midsection to prove it!!! How easy is *that*???

✓ Karate Kick: Don't know any martial arts? Doesn't matter! Just kick and punch. Start with one leg and kick in front of you 10-15 times. Then 10-15 with the next leg. Then punch in front of you 10-15 times with each arm. Do a few rounds of that. As you get better, add a different type of kick, even if you have to make one up because you don't know the moves officially. You'll get stronger, develop muscles and improve your mobility all at the same time. Just be careful not to kick or punch too hard in the beginning. I don't want you to hurt yourself or kick your legs from under you.

✓ Go skating: Whether you like to roller skate or roller blade, once you put on those wheels and get rolling, you'll start using muscles and joints that you may not have used in a while.

11. Weekend Warrior: Well, maybe not a "weekend" warrior, but definitely more warrior than the other suggestions. If you feel like you need a bit of a challenge, especially if you are typically more active anyway, you can try DVDs like P90X, Insanity, or the like. You can also pull out those old Billy Blanks discs. They are high intensity, high energy, and they are effective. But they are tough. If you choose to try one of these, go at your own pace until you get stronger. As you improve, you'll be able to continue at the pace of the people on the video.

12. Go to Boot Camp: If you've ever been in the military, known someone in the military or even watched *G.I. Jane*, you know that military PT workouts are rough but they train so that they can be in top condition in order to handle whatever obstacles come their way. If you want to train like the Army, Navy, Air Force or Marines, go on the internet and search for Military PT

workouts, then modify the workout to meet your current needs. As always, build your way up as you get stronger.

13. Boxing, MMA and Ultimate Fighting: Now, I know that this is a bit extreme, but keep it in mind as an option as you get stronger. It can always be a goal of yours. Start by stretching and developing your body, and develop into the next MMA champion!

CHAPTER 8

Get Some Sleep

CB ED

The best cure for insomnia is to get a lot of sleep – W.C. Fields

Sleep is one of the best, most rejuvenating methods of healing around. It has major anti-aging benefits. It can help reduce inflammation. It can help you think more clearly. And best of all, just like laughter, it is FREE!

When you are able to get sleep, especially if it's peaceful sleep, you are in a parasympathetic state. (Actually, the more you are in a parasympathetic state, the better quality sleep you will have.) See, the body has two main states: sympathetic and parasympathetic. Parasympathetic is also referred to as the "rest-and-digest" state of being, which is the exact opposite of your body's "fight-or-flight", or sympathetic state. In fight-or-flight, your body becomes more alert, your systems move a little faster, and your digestion slows or basically stops. All of this occurs so that you can focus all your energy on removing yourself from danger as quickly as possible. Needless to say that if your body is preparing to get out of danger, you won't be very calm or be able to rest very well.

In contrast, in the rest-and-digest state of being, digesting, healing, repair and growth are all processes that take quite a bit of energy to perform. In order for any of these to work fully, you must have adequate energy available   Sleep is important because this is the time your body takes to grow, heal, and repair. If you think about it, all three of those are a part of the same process. In each case, your body takes a tissue and remodels it in some way so as to have the tissue function the way that it should, which could include repairing damage or reshaping tissue because of growth that could occur from a newly introduced stressor (increased mobility, weight bearing exercise, etc.). Those processes require very high amounts of energy and resources, so in order for them to be done, and done maximally, you need to give them the time, space, and materials in order for them to take place. That time is during good sleep.

If you recall, young children always seem to sprout up overnight. That's because they pretty much do sprout overnight. And, when you become ill, you want to sleep much more often. Likewise, when you injure a body part, your doctor tells you to elevate it, secure it, stay off it, and get some rest. All of these examples fall in line with the same principle. Your body sends you the signal to rest and sleep so that you can do those things properly.

When you are in a stressful or dangerous situation, your body is preparing to remove you from harm's way. At that moment, internally there is no real difference between your having a 20 page paper due at 8am (that you hadn't started), or your running from the neighbor's dog that is chasing you. In either situation, your body is diverting a good bit of that energy and resources to your handling the situation. Conversely, when that happens you don't digest your food very well. Who needs to digest a steak when your body is trying not to become a steak?

You've heard it before "Sit down and eat your food"; "Don't eat on the go"; and "Don't go swimming right after you eat." All are sound advice. The main reason that these statements are around is because if you are doing other things, then there aren't as many resources of energy available for proper digestion. You also tend not to chew your food as well because you are not paying attention, running on autopilot, and rushing. So, even the beginning of digestion, the part that you have conscious control over, is not setting up the rest of the process to go as well as it could. If this happens chronically, you can get into a situation where you find that food begins to sit in your GI tract (digestive system) longer, and the food is not broken down as thoroughly.

Your system is not set up for maldigestion (poor and incomplete breakdown of food) or malabsorption (decreased ability for the proper nutrients to get into your body from your GI Tract), which is why your body will eventually malfunction (in part, because there aren't enough raw materials to help you function optimally). Couple all this with poor food choices – think Standard American Diet – that are very pro-inflammatory, highly processed, very low fiber and lacking many nutrients, and you have a system that is set up to fail from the start!

When you can work to get your body to relax more, you are in a better position to get quality sleep. When you are getting better sleep, you function better; you have more energy throughout the day; your memory improves; your body is less inflamed because it's healing better, and you are overall in a much better place in life.

Of course, there are other factors that determine the quality and quantity of sleep, just as there are other factors that determine how much energy you have and how healthy you are overall, but here are a few more to consider when you are trying to improve the quality and quantity of sleep:

1. Are you eating or drinking too much right before bed?
2. Is there too much on your mind to allow your brain to shut down?
3. Are you watching TV or listening to music that is too stimulating?
4. Are you reading materials that keep your mind working in overdrive?
5. Is it too hot or cold in your room?
6. Is your bed comfortable?
7. Are you going to bed too late and/or waking too early to allow yourself to get adequate hours of rest?
8. Is there too much light or noise around you?

This is just a short list of the things you can begin to consider when trying to create an environment that is more suitable for improved rest and sleep. For a complete list of ways to make your bedroom more sleep-encouraging, see Appendix A "Sleep Hygiene checklist"

ACTION PLAN:

1. Do 3-5 minutes of deep, relaxing breathing before going to bed. Focus on your breath and clear your mind of all the day's worries. Don't worry if it is more difficult to clear your mind in the beginning, just keep at it. The more you practice breathing deeply, the easier it will become. As 3-5 minutes gets easier, add an extra minute to your time. See Chapter 6, "Just Breathe," for more details on breathing exercises.

2. Meditate: Practice meditation and calming the mind. Turn on soothing sounds (music, nature sounds, etc.) that can help you relax and clear your mind. Work on emptying your mind of 'stuff' and filling it with calm, peace & serenity. This can definitely help you sleep more soundly

3. Drink warm herbal tea as the evening winds down. Begin to slow your pace, and start to focus on the beverage and your relaxation. Good herbs to try are chamomile, spearmint, tilia, orange blossoms, lemongrass, or valerian root. Any combination of these herbs or even a premixed sleep time blend will work well.

4. Place a pen and notebook near the head of your bed. Jot down any thoughts that may be running through your mind at the end of the night. Write all of those 'gotta dos', those 'don't forgets', or those brilliant ideas that always seem to come when your mind is trying to be free. By writing these down, you free your mind from having to remember them. This will give you hours of rest because you'll know that you won't forget.

5. Leave all electronics in another room, unless you are on-call at work. Then by all means, keep your phone or pager with you! There is really no need for the potential sleep disruption if it's not absolutely necessary. If you don't feel completely

comfortable leaving your gadgets in another room, at least turn them off (not sleep or silent, but OFF). This includes phones, tablets, iPads, laptops, desktops, and any other electronic gadget.

6. If you absolutely MUST have the phone in the room, turn the volume off, turn the vibrator off, and have the device face down so that you don't see the light in the middle of the night if it happens to come on. I'd hate to have a response to a Facebook post disturb your beauty rest!

7. Do some relaxing stretches before bed. Doing stretches will help ease muscle tension, increase blood flow to the muscles, and give your tissues more oxygen and nutrients which will allow them to heal better during the night while you rest.

8. Black it out: Put some dressing up over your windows to block out any light that may come through: street lights, porch lights, moon light, etc. Whatever light that may be peeking inside your window may be disrupting your sleep pattern. Melatonin, the sleep hormone produced in the body, is stimulated by darkness and turns to serotonin with light. By making your room extra dark (sheets, blankets, thick trash bags all work well), you are giving your endogenous melatonin greater opportunity to stick around and help you rest longer and better. BUT, don't forget to set your alarm. I'd hate for you to miss that important appointment because you were sleeping so well.

9. Take a relaxing bath before bed. The warm water will relax your muscles and decrease tension and stress. This will put you in a position to be more prepared for rest. For deeper relaxation, you can turn the lights off and light candles (the darkness will help to stimulate natural melatonin production), add Epsom Salt or Sea Salt (the magnesium and other minerals in the salts will relax muscles and feed tissues), and add essential oils to the water. Good essential oils to start out with are Lavender and Chamomile.

10. Check out Appendix A: Sleep Hygiene, for a checklist of things you can do to prepare your home and your body for slumber.

Sleep is the best meditation – *Dalai Lama*

CHAPTER 9

Wet My Whistle

Cß ßy

"Water is one of the most overlooked and important medicines of any time." – Dr. Steven Bailey, *The Fasting Diet*

The human body, just like the Earth, is made of more than 60-75% water. Water is necessary for the proper functioning of life, including temperature regulation, digestion, absorption and transportation of blood, hormones, and nutrients, metabolism and filtration just to name a few functions. We are constantly releasing water in the forms of sweat, breath, urine and stool. Even more water is lost, if we live in warmer, drier climates, during the summertime, engage in strenuous work or exercise and while at higher altitudes. The elderly, people on certain medications, and those that have a decreased sense of thirst may need even more water because they are at risk for quicker dehydration.

When you are dehydrated, you will usually feel thirsty. Thirst is the body's signal to increase water intake. What most people don't realize is that by the time they actually feel thirst, they are already in a state of dehydration.

If you are dehydrated enough or if there is chronic dehydration, you may put yourself at risk for headaches, fatigue, constipation, dry skin, electrolyte and pH imbalance, gall stones, kidney stones, heat exhaustion, and heat stroke. If you are working out and not replenishing water, your muscles will fatigue more quickly which will decrease your performance and increase your recovery time.

Dehydration is even said to be a main cause and contributor of jet lag! Who knew that the lack of otherwise ubiquitous water would have that kind of effect on the body?

There's a lot of conflicting information out there about how much water we should drink each day. Should we drink 8 eight oz. glasses? 10 glasses? Half our body weight? A gallon? Does coffee and soda count? Can water come from food? How big is a "cup"? (For the record, a 'cup' is 8 ozs; about the size of a medium or larger coffee mug.) So many questions that seem to have just as many answers. So many "expert" opinions. It's hard to know what information is right and what information is garbage. Hopefully, I can help you out with a little bit of practical information about water to help you get on track and stay hydrated.

First of all, you should be drinking a higher percentage of water than any other beverage. If you have more of other things than you have plain water, then you are probably more dehydrated than you think. Let's use this as an example: If you have 2 cups of coffee in the morning before breakfast, a large glass of orange juice with breakfast, a soda as a snack because you are thirsty, a soda for lunch with your meal, a large Starbuck's coffee as an afternoon pick-me-up, an energy drink in the evening and a cup of water with your dinner, then you are not drinking enough water. Even if you don't do percentages, the fact that you drank something 8 times and only one of those was water says that you didn't have enough water.

Second, most of the beverages you drink should have very few ingredients. The fewer the ingredients, especially those ingredients that can be pronounced and recognized, the better. You want to drink as few beverages with preservatives, colors, flavors (even 'natural flavors') and syrups as possible. These ingredients are not found in nature, they are created in a lab. Even the "natural" ingredients are not without some type of extensive processing that has to occur. The best bet is to try to drink things that are simple and that contain things that you know – water, pure fruit juices, sugar, herbs, honey, etc. You can't go wrong with this plan, especially if you are just starting out and trying to transition into drinking more healthy beverages.

Before I go any further, I'd like to clarify something. Above, I listed 'sugar' on the list of things to look for and drink. Know that I am not necessarily advocating that you drink a bunch of sugary drinks. What I am saying is that it is much better for your overall health and wellbeing if you just use sugar to sweeten your drinks than to use artificial sweeteners in the blue, yellow, or pink packets. There are several studies that report the harmful effects of those sweeteners. There is even a growing body of evidence that states that "diet" drinks that have artificial sweeteners may cause more weight gain, not less. These are definitely not things you want in your body. So, if it's a choice between a white packet of sugar and a packet of another color, go for the sugar. Eventually, your goal should be to decrease the amount of sweeteners you use, natural or artificial, so that you can decrease that caloric burden on your body and begin to enjoy the true taste of the foods that you are eating.

Next, if you can't see through the drink, it's probably more dehydrating to the body than hydrating. Dark sodas, thick, sugary Kool-Aid, Fruit Cocktails/Drinks (those with very little real juice in them) are all very concentrated. Even the "100% Fruit Juices" are very concentrated and can point the body in the wrong direction of hydration if you drink enough of them.

The sweeter the beverage, the more dehydrating it will be on the inside of your body. If everything you drink has to be very sweet – with loads of sugar, or honey, or the artificial stuff – then your body will have to work to make it the correct osmolarity (concentration of water vs. what's dissolved in it). In order to achieve the correct osmolarity your body takes the water that is in your cells in order to dilute your beverage. When it does, it will basically leave those cells thirsty. Too much sugar, honey, or sweetener, once inside the body, will require extra resources for the body to balance it out. In order for the sugary beverages to cause less damage and be properly processed your body will have to add extra water and nutrients. If you aren't taking in much water then your body will take what it can, which will leave other areas starving for water. Then those other areas will steal water from nearby tissues, which will then steal from the tissues next to them... and the vicious cycle has begun.

One way you can help this process is by decreasing the amount of sweeteners you have in your drinks. For some of you, this may be much more difficult than for others. But trust me, the more you do it, the more your taste buds will adapt, and you'll begin to enjoy, and even crave the refreshing taste of the less sweetened drinks!

The last strategy that I'll introduce is to make more of your beverages at home. The more you begin to make your own, the more control you have over what goes into those beverages. You will also have a greater opportunity to be more creative and mix your own blends. By doing this, you may find something that you've never had before and that makes you feel like a superhero!! You never know.

ACTION PLAN:

Here are some ways to increase your water consumption and get rehydrated. For other ideas, please refer to chapter 13, "Let's Eat!", for different beverage recipes.

1. Drink a bottle (16 oz.) or a large glass of water as soon as you wake up in the morning. If you don't mind room temperature water, then you can have this water sitting by your bedside. This way it is readily available to you when you wake up.
2. If you must drink sodas, drink those that have real sugar instead of artificial sweeteners. Please know that I am by no means advocating drinking sodas, nor am I saying that sodas with sugar are healthy. What I'm saying is that if you absolutely must have soda, please choose one with potentially the least amount of burden on your body.

3. For every amount of soda you drink, have an equal amount of water. A can of soda is 10oz. Drink at least 10oz of water either before or after your soda.
4. Make it visible: If you have a desk at work, put a large cup, water bottle, or jar in front of you. You want to have something sitting nearby that you can reuse. Try drinking at least one of the large cups or water bottles the first half of the workday.
5. Try drinking that same amount of water during the second half of your workday.
6. Drink a large glass of water as soon as you come home from work. Do this as soon as you walk in the door.
7. Drink a large glass of water before you go to bed. If you have trouble with waking in the middle of the night to urinate, then try drinking the water a few hours before bed so that you are less likely to have to get up in the night.
8. Add different fruit to your jar or cup of water. Great fruit to start with are lemons and limes, but don't stop there. Expand your horizons. Try adding orange and grapefruit slices. You can also consider adding kiwi or strawberries. How about a bit of frozen fruit? Add some blackberries, blueberries or a berry bend to the water. How about melon cubes? Be adventurous!
9. Add vegetables or herbs! Cucumber slices are extremely refreshing. Celery can be amazing at adding electrolytes. Carrot shreds added to water and allowed to sit overnight in the fridge can be a real Caribbean treat. Adding herbs like fresh peppermint, basil, or rosemary can be great additions and adds medicinal benefits to help you along your healing journey.
10. Get the family involved: Have other members of the family come up with flavor combinations for your beverages. They will be much more willing to make changes like the ones you have made, if they are actively involved in the decision making and creative process, even if it's in this very small way to begin with.
11. Make it Fresh Daily: Make a fresh fruit/veggie/herbal infused water each day. That can be your family's beverage for the day. By making a large container each day, you can monitor what

your family is drinking (or at least a portion of it what they drink) throughout the day.

12. Dilute your juice: When drinking a juice, begin adding ¼ volume water and the rest juice. After you've done that for a little while and have gotten used to it, start adding a bit more water until it's half and half. Eventually, you can get yourself to the point that you are drinking ¾ glass water, ¼ glass juice and ultimately water with just a splash of your favorite juice for a little touch of flavor.

13. Begin brewing and drinking more herbal teas. Teas are wonderful because each herb has amazing health benefits and they have different flavors. It's easy to mix & match and change the taste. You can also get a dose of herbal 'medicine' with each cup. How about that? Every sip can go toward helping improve some aspect of your health.

14. Make a conscious effort to eat more fresh, raw fruit and veggies. Each bite is not only filled with vitamins, minerals, chlorophyll, fiber and phytonutrients (nutrients unique to plants) but it is also full of life giving, life sustaining water. You're in essence chewing your water. Isn't that cool?!

15. There's an App for that: Find and download an app on your Smartphone that will remind you to drink more water and can help you track how much water you've already had. Use your technology to improve your health!

16. Eat your water: Making homemade soup, without too much salt of course, can be a great way to increase your hydration! Making soup that has lots of fresh veggies and herbs on a regular basis can really help you get more water in while increasing your nutrient intake. Be careful not to add too many artificial ingredients (packets of seasonings that have artificial ingredients, preservatives, colors, etc.) to your soup.

17. Have a coconut: Coconut water is like nature's "Gatorade." It contains the right amount of natural sugars, electrolytes and other nutrients to help rehydrate and rebalance a body. Coconut water is a great drink to have on a hot day, and it's also

good to use during and after workouts. Several companies sell it, so you want to look for the brands that only have "coconut water" listed in the ingredients. You can also try cracking open your own nut for that on-the-beach refreshment.

Remember not to overwhelm yourself. Go as far as you can and do as much as you can sustain. Pick one or two of these to do. Try them out for a few weeks. Get used to it. Then add or try something new. Make it easy. **Make it FUN!**

If you have any health conditions that caused your physician to restrict the amount of fluids you drink each day, follow the recommendations of your physician. In those cases, drinking more water and other fluids may be more detrimental to your health than beneficial. Always discuss those and other changes with your Licensed Naturopath, MD, or other licensed health care practitioner before making these suggested changes. In this case, you might just try improving the quality of your fluids so that you are drinking the best, most beneficial and healing fluids available to you.

CHAPTER 10

Take a Commercial Break

 C8 80

"When in doubt, go on vacation" – Author Unknown

In the Western world, we live in an always-on-the-go, never-take-a-break, I'll-Sleep-when-I-die type of environment. This is thought to be great for productivity (though that's really questionable), but it's not so great for the health and wellbeing of the individuals doing it.

In the early days of civilization, before technology and fast living, we lived in forests, mountains, plains, and deserts. In each community everyone had a particular task to do in order to maintain the functionality of the family and community as a whole. There were those that hunted, those that farmed, and those that worked in the community in other capacities. Every now-and-then a threat would present itself – Lions and Tigers and Bears... Oh MY! – When that happened, they'd either have to defend themselves against the threat (fight) or they'd have to run as fast as they could in order to avoid becoming the next meal (flight). Once the threat of danger had passed, they'd take a deep breath, assess the damages, and get back to business. No more threat. No more stress, at least not until the next threat came along. This is how humans were designed. This is how the Fight-or-Flight response is supposed to work. It is supposed to turn on when you are in imminent danger and turn off when the danger has subsided.

This is called the Stress Response. You know it. You've experienced it. It's what happens when the neighbor's dog gets out of the gate and decides that your butt looks like dinner. It's what makes your heart start racing, your blood move faster in your vessels, your hearing become more acute, your pupils dilate, you start breathing faster, and your adrenaline starts pumping. All of this happens so that you get more blood, fuel, and oxygen to your muscles, allowing you to run faster or fight harder. Your fight-or-flight response, also known as the sympathetic response, is designed to get you out of danger quickly.

What you may not realize is that those everyday stressors in life, both big and small, are treated the same way internally. Whether you are in rush hour traffic, trying to meet a deadline at work, paying bills or making dinner for a hungry, impatient family, the internal response is the same. Your body doesn't know the difference. All your body knows is that it needs to get you out of danger quickly!

Through technological, industrial, and scientific advances we have gotten to a point where we are more 'on' than 'off'. The Stress Response has almost no time to shut off and reset. We wake up early to cram for that test that we didn't study for. Then we rush to get dressed. We go to the corner drive-thru to grab an extra-large coffee (with extra espresso and a few pumps of the sweet goodness) and a sugary snack. We get stuck in morning traffic and yell at the person that just cut us off. We take the test, five minutes late, all the while freaking out because we didn't get to study that last section of notes (and of COURSE it's the biggest part of the test). We then rush off to work and deal with the cranky clients. The boss demands that everything happens immediately. Evening traffic is even worse than morning traffic. Then there are bills, violent TV shows, family... it never ends. We more often than not, wake up the next morning (if we're able to get any sleep at all) and repeat the same scenario. Each of those situations alone is treated as imminent danger within the body. Each one causes the same chemical cascade that will cause you to try to either fight or run (theoretically speaking). Put them all together in that string of events, and do that every day for weeks, months or even years and you can see how it can wear you out from the inside.

For optimal health we need to create some structured downtime within our hectic lives. I'm not just talking about the occasional trip to Hawaii. There needs to be enough "off" time to help you sustain and rejuvenate yourself from all of your 'on' time. Without having that downtime, you create an internal environment that is much more susceptible to fatigue, exhaustion, headaches and memory loss, aging, mistakes and even disease. No matter how productive you want or need to be, the fact of the matter is that you can never be as effective as you are when you are well rested.

You have to take commercial breaks. You have to take time off from your regularly scheduled program so that you can get other things done. Just like on TV, where you have regular 30 second commercials, 1 minute commercials, and the occasional 30-60 minute infomercial, you have to take time out to check out some different things before you refocus on that task at hand.

In order to obtain and maintain health, you should take those long, 1-2 week Exotic Island vacations as often as you and your family can afford. But, let's face it, for the average American, it isn't very realistic to take one every year. For many people, it may only be every 2-3 years or even 2-3 times in a life time. It's usually more feasible to take a vacation to another part of the country, to an amusement park, a national monument, or maybe even a nearby beach. Even more common is a mini-vacation or trip to a friend or relative's house.

When it comes to your health, you should begin to think about taking mini-mini-vacations more often than not. The more you can do it, the more likely you are to handle a day's stress with grace. Here's how you can work it into your life:

ACTION PLAN:

1. Breathe: Start by doing breathing exercises for 5 minutes every morning. Sit in a chair, feet flat on the floor, palms on your thighs, back straight but relaxed. Close your eyes and slowly

inhale for a count of four. Hold your breath for a two count then exhale slowly for a count of four. Set a stopwatch (the one on your phone will do just fine) or an alarm clock so that you can focus on breathing and not worry about the amount of time that's passed. Once you've gotten this down, check out Chapter 6, "Just Breathe", for more varieties of ways to incorporate better breathing into your day.

2. Go to your Exotic place: If you ever watched the movie 'Collateral' with Jamie Foxx and Tom Cruise, you know that Foxx's character was a cab driver. One thing that he did that really stuck with me was that he had a picture of an exotic island in his car's visor. He said that when things got hectic he would look at it and go on vacation several times a day. I think that we should all do that! Find a photo of some exotic land that you've either visited in the past or would like to visit. Print or cut this picture out and post it somewhere that you can see it often. This may be the visor of your car, on the wall behind the desk at your cubicle, or on the refrigerator at home. Wherever it is, make sure that you can get to it often so that you can escape for a brief moment into that serene place. Look at it for several minutes, a few times a day. Think only of that place. Think about the way it makes you feel, and all the sights and sounds you expect to experience while there. Allow your imagination to get creative. Enjoy your vacation... with a smile.

3. Ground Yourself: We often forget, or don't realize that we are electrical beings. Electricity, "energy," protons and electrons make us run. Just like any other thing that runs on electricity, we need to be grounded. Take some time to (literally) reconnect with the Earth around you. Walk barefoot in the grass, sit under a tree, put a blanket on the ground and lay down – or just lay on the ground itself, sit amongst the flowers, hug a huge tree... all these activities can help you recharge. The earth beneath you will act like the third prong of an outlet. It doesn't have to be much at first. It just takes a little bit of conscious effort, but it can make all the difference in the world

to help relax you, calm you, and help you put your life in better perspective. Check Chapter 11, "Get Grounded," for more ideas.

4. Take the scenic route: every so often, take a different route to or from work. Pay attention to all the sights around you – trees, houses, buildings, mountains, sunset, etc. Begin to actually pay attention to things and learn something new about your neighborhood and your city. You'll be amazed at all the things you will 'discover' when you start to look at familiar settings with unfamiliar eyes.

5. Play with kids: Take time out to actually have fun with your little people. It doesn't have to take up a lot of your time and energy.   The most important thing is to give them your undivided attention and that you are present in the moment. Take the focus away from your problems. You can read to them, play pitch-and-catch, have a hula hoop contest, color, talk about your childhood or make up fairy tales. It really doesn't matter. Just spend some quality time with them and learn to smile as much as they do. You will also build a much stronger bond that they will cherish for many years to come.

6. Have a lunch or dinner date with the spouse / significant other. Focus on one another. Learn something new about each other. Only talk about good things. Make each other laugh. Play footsie. Fall in love again... every day!

7. Go Play: Do something fun and silly. Do cartwheels in the park. Go play paintball. Ride the train at the park and make train sounds ("chooooo choooooooooo") while you wave at all the people you pass by. Get on the swings and try to kick the sky. Have a water gun sneak attack fight with the neighbors (the fun neighbors, not the ones that will call the cops or shoot you with their glock or anything). Re-learn to be silly.

8. Find a hobby: Start doing that thing that you've been wanting to do for the last few years. Take a dance class. Learn to play the piano. Start to do needle point. Pick up a camera and take pictures of your city. Do Qi Gong. Plant that garden. Learn to

play ping pong. Whatever it is, make time to learn it and do it regularly.

9. Read a book: Pick a book that has nothing to do with your line of work. Let the book take you away. Begin to use your imagination again!

10. Go to the movies: Go to a matinee so that the theater is relatively empty (it's cheaper anyway). Maybe even go to the $2 / discount Movie Theater, and watch an older release. It doesn't matter. Just go.

11. Take naps: Most people don't rest very much anyway, so begin to take naps when you can. Remember how much energy children have after a nap?? Try to recapture some of your own energy with a 10 minute power nap in the middle of the day. Call it a siesta!

12. Go to the park and read: Carry a good book with you. Put it in your purse, in your car, or in your backpack. When you get a free moment (or when you take a free moment), sit in a quiet place in a park or on a beautifully landscaped area and take it all in. Then pull out your book and read a chapter or two. It doesn't have to be a lot. Just a bit to get you engrossed in a story for a few minutes and allow your imagination to take over. Once you've read that chapter or two come back to reality, look at your surroundings again. Appreciate its beauty and serenity. Now, go on your way…. With a smile!

13. Laugh!!! Laughter is magical. It can instantly diffuse a situation and release pinned up tension. If you need suggestions on ways to laugh more, check out Chapter 4, "What's So Funny?"

14. Learn to meditate: a 10-15 minute quiet meditation session can be as refreshing as a 1 hour nap. The more you do it, the better you get at it. So, learn how to do it and then do it often. Be silent.

15. Make a paper airplane! I recently helped a friend practice their public speaking skills by critiquing their presentation on making a paper airplane. It reminded me that I hadn't made one in FOREVER!! So, I made my airplane and it was fun. It didn't take

long, it was inexpensive, I had fun, and I recycled it! What more could you ask for??

True silence is the rest of the mind, and is to the spirit what sleep is to the body, nourishment and refreshment. – William Penn

CHAPTER 11

Get Grounded

Cʒ ꝏ

"Feel the Force!" – Yoda

I recently went to a lecture by one of my former instructors, Dr. Matt Baral. He was talking about the affect Nature has on the health of humans. After listening to this lecture, I decided that I must add this chapter to the book (even though I had pretty much finished the book). It was a powerful message that he shared with us and I felt that I'd be doing you a disservice not to pass my own version of that information on to you.

During the talk, he brought up several very interesting research studies from all over the world that showed that people in general do much better when they are in nature, around nature, or even look at pictures of nature. As long as there was some connection to nature, there was a benefit to health experienced. Here are some examples of what he presented:

- ✓ People are more likely to spend more money, even on the exact same items, in malls that have trees.
- ✓ Children that are in a classroom with plants, even if the plants are in the back of the room where the children can't see them very easily, were more attentive and had fewer visits to the nurse than those that were in classrooms without plants.
- ✓ Elders that have gardens to care for or fish to look at have less cognitive decline, they eat more, and they tend to wander less. They are also less aggressive towards their caregivers.

- ✓ Salivary cortisol levels decreased in people sitting in nature for 20 minutes. This means that sitting in a park or amongst trees or some other natural setting can help decrease the body's stress response.
- ✓ Contact with nature cuts the health discrepancy between poor and rich people in half. What this means is that when poor people are in nature on a regular basis they are less sick. This causes the differences in their health/healthcare and that of rich people to be much less.
- ✓ There is significantly less dementia when elders spend time in nature.
- ✓ Earthing helps decrease blood viscosity. This means that laying or sleeping on the ground, or even sitting with your bare feet on the earth for a length of time can act as a natural blood thinner.
- ✓ Earthing during sleep was found to improve sleep quality, and reduce pain and stress. That's to say that connecting to the earth (grounding yourself) while sleeping can help you be in less pain, eliminate some stress, and help you sleep better – which will improve your overall health even more.
- ✓ Earthing may help regulate the Endocrine (hormonal) and Nervous systems. These are the top two systems in the body to regulate everything else in the body.

All of that from just connecting to, caring for, being in the presence of or just focusing on nature? Who knew?!

Well, it really shouldn't come as a surprise. Humans, as are all living creatures, are electrical beings. We have "energy" that allows us to survive, live and thrive.

When Earth and the universe were created (or evolved, if that's your belief system), it was done in a way that connected everything to everything else. There was harmony. Everything was interconnected. The Earth and Soil were where we got out food. The trees provided shelter for countless animals and insects. Humans exhaled carbon dioxide that the trees could then use. They then took in that carbon dioxide and released oxygen, their waste product, so that we can breathe. When animals release waste (urinate or defecate) it goes back to the earth, ages, and becomes fertilizer for the plants. Even when we die, we go back to earth and fertilize the soil so that the cycle of life can continue (ashes to ashes, dust to dust).

It is modern society that has driven us farther and farther away from our connection to earth and nature. It is also modern society that seems to be driving us to decline in health, especially those "diseases of lifestyle" (those that are caused by, or significantly contributed to, by the way we live).

One of the key components to moving back towards health may be as simple as going outside for a little while each day because we now know that connection to nature can do all of the following:

- ❖ Improve attention span and focus
- ❖ Regulate our immune system
- ❖ Decrease stress
- ❖ Improve sleep
- ❖ Positively affect the cardiovascular system by decreasing blood viscosity and improving blood pressure
- ❖ Improve brain function
- ❖ Decease cognitive decline and dementia as we age
- ❖ And improve overall health

Why wouldn't we want to do something so simple, cheap, and possibly lifesaving? Here are some ways that you can increase your connection to the earth on a daily basis.

ACTION PLAN:

- Cut out, purchase, or print a picture of some natural setting that moves you. Put it somewhere that will make it easily seen on a regular basis. At least twice a day, look at it for at least 5 minutes. Focus solely on it and nothing else. Escape to that place and imagine what's around you. Immerse yourself in all the sights, sounds, smells and feelings of that piece of paradise. Once you get comfortable doing this, increase it to 3, 4, 5, etc. times a day. Go there as often as you need to in order to recharge and get away from the stressors of the day.

- Before work, during lunch, and/or after getting home go out to some patch of grass and take off your shoes. Put your feet on the ground for 5 minute (be careful not to step in an ant pile or any dog doody!) Just relax and focus on the ground beneath your feet. Is it cold? Wet? Dry? Is it soft? Are there prickly pears sticking your feet? Just take note of it all.

- On your drive to/from work, notice if there are any parks or park-like places in the area. When you have the time, go there, find a secluded place, and just take a seat. Now breathe. Even better, bring a book or some relaxing music (nothing too fast, heavy, wordy, bass filled, etc.). Focus all your attention on that for the next 20 minutes. Just read your book or listen to the relaxing music, and let your attention be drawn to that and the nature that surrounds you.

- If you have a hobby – knitting, crocheting, playing an instrument, making origami swans, etc. – do it while sitting outside on a bench under a big'ole tree (or a big'ole bush if you live in the desert).

- Go to the local park (the bigger the better) or a forest, mountain or creek. Wander around for at least an hour. Follow a trail, or maybe follow the path of the creek. Leave your phone in your car, or at least put it away and don't access it until you get back to "reality." Be sure to turn the ringer off if you keep your phone with you (or better yet, turn off the phone) while you are on your trip. Make it a point to discover, explore and 'get lost' in nature. Touch the trees. Smell the flowers. Look at the insects. Hear the rustling of the leaves and grass. Immerse yourself in your surroundings.

- Take a weekend road trip to a national park, beach or a mountainous area.

- Grow a plant, preferably something edible, but ultimately grow anything that you feel like growing (as long as it's legal!) If you don't want to buy a plant, get a cutting from a friend or family member. Alternately, you can just take a seed from a fruit in your refrigerator and put it in some dirt. That way, you can watch it grow through all of its stages. If you'd like to take it a bit further, take photos at each stage of growth. You can even take pictures daily to document your 'experiment.'

- Plant a garden: Grow some flowers. Grow some food. Grow ANY food or a combination of food and flowers. The size of the garden is up to you and the amount of space you have. It can be a fresh herb garden in a small pot or two in your kitchen near a window, or a salad garden in a larger pot on your porch or balcony. You can even do a square foot garden in the yard or a flower garden in front of the house. Just pick a space, find a pot that will accommodate your needs and plant some stuff!!

- Keep a small blanket in the trunk of your car. When you get (or make) an opportunity, have your lunch outside picnic style. Don't make a big deal out of it or you'll be much less likely to do it. Just grab any blanket or sheet that you don't mind getting dirty, fold it up and put it in the trunk. The next time you go out for carry-out, just stop somewhere and sit out to eat.

- Go camping: Sleep outside for a night or two. Sleep under the stars, away from street lights, electric wires and electromagnetic waves, Wi-Fi, and all things electronic. Allow your body to be free of all the "noise", seen and unseen, that you are bombarded with on a daily basis.

- Purchase an Earthing mat: Earthing companies have mats, sheets, pillowcases, pads, throws, etc. that tap into the electromagnetic 'grounding' potential of the earth. By using these products with as much skin contact as possible, you are allowing the earth to realign your energy/electrons. If you use them while you sleep, you are getting the added benefit of allowing the product and the earth to help you sleep better. As we know, getting a better quality sleep will rejuvenate you more completely. There's no better time for realignment and healing than when you sleep. Why not use something that may help you sleep longer, deeper and better?

Whatever you decide to do, know that you're doing it to get more connected to the Earth, to yourself, and to have more overall balance mentally, physically emotionally and spiritually.

CHAPTER 12

You Are What You Eat

CS ∂O

You are what you eat, so don't be fast, cheap, easy, or fake. – Facebook Meme

It's time to talk about food. This is probably the most important part of this book after Chapter 3, "Change Your Seat, Change Your Life." Most of us don't realize just how important food is in the quality of our lives and in our health. No matter what society or culture we come from, food plays a pivotal role. We use it to help define and express our customs, traditions and rituals. There are foods that we must eat and those that we must avoid according to certain spiritual beliefs. When we celebrate, mourn, or meet we always have food present. There are cities, towns and industries built around certain foods. These are the things that most of us realize.

What many of us don't realize is how health, good or bad, is built around the foods we eat. Our bodies are made up of chemicals, nutrients and molecules. Our foods are made up of chemicals, nutrients, and molecules. Every time we eat, drink and inhale there are chemical reactions that occur. It's what keeps us alive. It's what keeps us moving. How **well** you are moving or how truly 'alive' you are depends on several things, many of which are outlined here in this book. The better quality the food, beverages, air and thoughts that enter your body, the better the quality of your body. Like they say, 'You are what you eat.'

Here are a couple examples that will hopefully help you put things in better perspective. You like to drive cars. Maybe you like to drive fast. Maybe you are a race car driver as your profession or hobby. No matter how much you love cars; there are certain things that you must have. You know that you want a car that's eye catching and beautiful. The car you drive is an extension of you so it should be aesthetically appeasing to you (and possibly to those around you). The reality is that no matter how good this car looks, if it doesn't run well, it isn't worth nearly as much because it can't function the way it's supposed to. If it can't get you from point A to point B in a timely fashion, what's the use in having it, right? So, you make sure that your car gets regular checks, you bring it in when there are lights blinking on the dash or something starts to buzz. You have the fluid levels checked and changed as often as necessary and you only give it the best quality materials (oil, gas, tires, hoses and belts) because you know that anything less will decrease your car's performance. If you do give your car less than optimal products, you already know that it may run slowly or stall; or there may be some sputtering or dragging. The car may make any number of other interesting noises. This is just not what you want from your valued vehicle.

Your body is very similar. YOU are a high performance vehicle. You are resilient but still sensitive to everything that is around you and everything that goes inside you. The lower quality fuel you put in your body, the lower your performance output. The more poor quality food, drink, air, thoughts, etc. that you put into your system, the more likely you are to move slowly, to stall, sputter and drag. That's just not what you want from your valued body.

Unlike the car though, you cannot just change out parts that are worn, broken, or cracked. You can't just go to the doctor's office, pick out the parts you want and get all new tubes, an engine or batteries in an hour. It just doesn't happen that way. Of course there is plastic surgery, stints, transplants and other procedures, but they are not available to most people and they are (or at least should) only available to those that really need it. On top of that, they are very costly procedures not only financially, but in the time and energy it takes to heal and move forward. In essence, it's something that you want to avoid as much as possible.

Even though you can't just change out your parts at will, the beauty and miracle of you is that your body can heal. When given the right materials and the right amount of time, you can rebuild an entirely new you. You can restore, renew, and reconstruct your entire body when you have the right conditions. You just have to make the right materials available to your cells when they need them. That's where your food comes in.

Your food, the stuff that you put in your body 3-6 times a day, has a HUGE effect on you. Your food can be the best, safest, most powerfully healing medicine that you ever have. Conversely, your food can be the slowest form of death by poisoning that there is. Don't believe me? Think about it. Is there something that you eat that gives you a headache, makes you sleepy, gives you acid reflux, makes your nose run, causes you to sneeze, give you a tummy ache, or raises your blood pressure? These are warning signals by the body. Your body is telling you that something is just not right. The more you ignore those signals, the more you are giving your body an opportunity to continue on a path of destruction. In other words, you are encouraging a slow, insidious death. On the other hand, there are foods that give you energy when you eat them. Not like hyped up, caffeine laden, 5-hour-energy type of energy. I'm talking about that "I feel really good and can get so much done right now" type energy. There are foods that actually make your tummy feel good and make you feel relaxed. There are foods that can fill you up and *not* put you to sleep. These are good foods. Foods that are more healing than destroying.

It's unfortunate that we are not a culture that teaches about eating real food, eating foods that are in season and eating food that will improve life and preserve health. These are our circumstances. This is what we were given. We are not taught how to have a healthy relationship with food. Most of us don't even realize things like fresh produce will usually have dirt on it. As a matter of fact, we think of dirt as this nasty, bug-y, germ infested stuff that is totally gross and will kill us (or at least make us very sick) if we eat any of it. I've met children and heard of children that have never seen cauliflower, don't know what a whole, fresh tomato looks like, or who don't even know that fruit are supposed to have seeds (which is part of what defines it as a fruit).

What we are taught is how to "live to eat", instead of eating to live. The message that food can help us through tough times is always around. Food becomes a crutch, much like many drugs, in helping us deal with the present situation without us actually dealing with the present situation. The way we live our lives discourages foods prepared fresh in the kitchen, family meals at the table, or anything that takes longer than the 3 minutes it usually takes the microwave to beep. Most of our food comes from across the country or even overseas (I still don't understand why there is Salmon from Scotland in the stores. SCOTLAND!!) The produce is picked before it has had a chance to ripen and then it's sprayed with chemicals to help keep bugs away, keep it from molding, and keep it from sprouting. While that may be a great financial move for the corporation that sells the product, this is not a very good option for our individual health.

Our meats are raised in less than optimal conditions where the animals are made to grow by modifying their genes and giving them hefty amounts of growth hormones making them too big too fast for their limbs to carry them. They are being injected with antibiotics to prevent and treat infections that tend to occur because of the unnatural foods they are fed and living quarters that they live in. The animals are also not allowed to roam free and eat the foods that they are naturally meant to eat. All of these factors change the quality, taste and health profile of the food that ends up on our dinner plates.

Looking at all this stuff, you may be tempted to ask "What's the point? I don't have any control over any of that." On the contrary!!! You have all the control. And the point is that the more you take control over what goes on your dinner plate, the more the supermarkets, restaurants and larger corporations will have to take note and start catering to you and others like you. It's the power of the dollar. It's supply and demand. You ever notice how some items are found in grocery stores in some neighborhoods and not others? Think about how some "ethnic" foods have a spot on a shelf in one store but across town the entire store is 'ethnic.' Or how one store will have certain varieties, colors, and name brands of some products and some will only have generic or common brands. That's supply and demand at work.

Once you start to make changes personally, you can influence those around you. They then influence those around them, and so on. Eventually, you have entire communities making changes for the better. Once that happens, businesses must take notice, especially if they want to stay in business. And THAT's how you build stronger, healthier communities!!! Now, let's get ready to change the world!!

CHANGE YOUR MIND:

There are certain mindsets that need to be overcome first when making changes to the way you eat. Because food is so ingrained in the way we live, it can be difficult to think differently about it, but it can be done. As long as you are alive, you can make changes to your food choices and improvements to your health.

> ➤ Breakfast food at breakfast time: One of the most common comments that I hear is that you've got to eat breakfast foods during breakfast time. We consider breakfast foods to be pancakes, waffles, French toast, Pop Tarts, cold cereals… and meat. This is the mindset that persists mostly in North American and Western cultures. Know that it's ok to have savory (non-sweet) meals for breakfast. It's even ok to have a hefty dose of veggies in the morning!
> ➤ "Diet sodas are ok": Many people think drinking soda is fine as long as it's diet because it has no calories, right? Not exactly. More and more research is coming out proving that not only are

diet sodas *not* a better choice than regular sodas, but in fact they can actually lead to some pretty hefty deficiencies and illnesses. Diet drinks can lead to increased weight gain. They create greater hunger which leads to eating more food (which is usually not going to be veggies, but some highly processed, high carbohydrate, box food). If you absolutely MUST have a soda, it is better to get one sweetened with real sugar. The better option is one that is sweetened with stevia or honey. The absolute best option is to not drink them at all.

➤ "If it was good for my mother/father/grandparents then it's good enough for me": There are several things wrong with this statement. For one, the food we are currently eating is not the same quality as the food our parents and grandparents ate. The nutritional profile has been shown to be much worse. The food comes from further away and is usually much more processed, genetically modified, and altered. Second, keep in mind that elders were generally much more physically active in their younger years than we are now. They didn't have the technology that we rely on and take for granted so they had to do much more stuff on their own. They had to get in there and use 'elbow grease' to get things done. Lastly, keep in mind that there were still diseases. What they ate could actually have been, and probably was, contributing to their disease processes but the fact that they were more active and the food was generally a better quality probably helped to keep them from being as sick as we are now.

➤ "Isn't food meant to be enjoyed?" ABSOLUTELY!!! Here's the thing. Corporations spend a lot of money to have scientists create the perfect taste, texture, and smell combinations which are usually artificial. We've gotten desensitized to the true flavor of foods so that it's much more difficult to like real foods. But that can all change, and it WILL! We are going to learn how to enjoy real food and then we are going to enjoy the awesome benefits and the way you feel when you eat those real foods!

➢ "I just don't have the time to think about, prepare and cook food": You know, just because you decide not to focus on something or not make it a priority, doesn't mean that it will go away. Trust me. I've tried. Every now-and-then things will miraculously disappear but usually, it just festers and gets worse. You may not be ready right now, and that's ok. It's your decision. Just be aware that it's possible that things may continue to progress in the same direction that they were going if you don't make a certain change to the way you eat. They may get worse before they get better. When you decide that something is a priority in your life, you will make time for it. Once you make time for it, it becomes easier and doesn't take much time or effort. You just have to make the decision to carve out some time and space for it in your life.

"A crust eaten in peace is better than a banquet partaken in anxiety" - Aesop

ACTION PLAN:

1. Eat In Peace: When you are about to eat a meal or snack make a concerted effort to sit in a quiet peaceful place without distraction. The more calm and relaxed your body is when you eat, the better you will digest your food. This will help the overall process of eating for health become even more profound.

2. Know why you are eating your food: Are you really hungry, or do you just feel like eating? Could you be thirsty and not realize it? Are you eating because you are sad, lonely, need consoling? Are you bored? Are you eating out of habit or because something is sitting there and you can't avoid it? Pay attention to the 'why'. Begin to only eat when you are hungry and for no other reason. If you are eating because of an emotion – boredom, anger, sadness, loneliness – then try to find another way to console yourself and fill your time. Go for a walk. Call a

friend. Go to a matinee. Read a book. Find a more productive way to handle your emotions and develop a healthier relationship with food.

3. Do some Push-Backs: I come from the land of great food. I know what it feels like to keep eating because the food is just so good that you don't want the experience to end. But you want to develop self-control when you eat. Learn to pay attention to your body so that you can actually know when you are about 80% full, and then stop. Push yourself back from the table (push-backs). If you have food left on your plate, wrap it up and save it for the next meal. Usually it tastes even better when the food and spices have had time to sit for a little while anyway!

4. Drink some water: When you get hungry, drink a large glass of water before you actually sit down to your meal. Sometimes, the hunger sensation that you feel is really thirst. If you drink water 15-30 minutes before you eat, you may be able to eat less because you are actually giving your body what it really wants, water. If that doesn't help, at least you'll be a bit more hydrated.

5. Eat at least 2 servings (1 cup) of cooked veggies every day. If you already eat that, increase whatever you do eat by a cup. Vary the types of vegetables you eat. Good choices are Broccoli, cauliflower, spinach, kale, chard, kohlrabi, squash, artichoke, eggplant, sprouts, celery, greens and okra. Of course there is more out there. The choices are endless!! Also remember not to overcook your veggies! You want your veggies to still have the same vibrant color and crunch that it had when it was raw. The more it's cooked, the fewer nutrients present.

6. Eat at least 2 servings of *raw* veggies each day (a serving is 1 cup). This is different from #5 because this is focused on eating it in its freshest form. Raw veggies and fruit have enzymes and nutrients that tend to be better for digestion, often times absorbed better in the body and offers more to the cells in the way of nutrients. They are literally 'living' foods. If you want to

live more and have a more vibrant life, you want to eat more live, vibrant foods.

7. Eat at least one serving of fresh fruit everyday: If you already eat some daily, add one more serving. A serving size is 1 small apple, 1 pear, or ½ cup of melons, berries, pineapple, papaya, mango, or any other fruit. Vary the fruit that you eat. Try a new fruit that you've never had before. Experiment and widen your selections.

8. Decrease your Meat: We've gotten to the point where meat and protein make up the majority of our meals. The rest of the meal being high carbohydrate foods and very little produce. We think that if we don't have a quarter pound, half pound, or pound of meat on the plate that we won't get the adequate amount of nutrients, especially protein, that we need to function. Know that this is absolutely false! You don't need to have steak, bacon, chicken, ribs, and turkey at every meal in order to survive. In fact, it has been show in numerous studies that too much of these foods can actually lead to more problems like inflammation, slowed digestion, and an increased risk for cancers! Adding more plant foods – nuts, seeds, beans, lentils, and leafy greens – can give you quite a bit of protein. This plant protein is often easier for the body to process and has more nutrients that will benefit, cleanse, and heal the body. Try having no more than 3oz of meat at any given meal. That is roughly the size of a deck of cards or a hockey puck.

9. Meatless Mondays: One day a week – it doesn't have to be Mondays, but it does have a certain ring to it, doesn't it?? – eat all your meals without any meat, or other animal products. You can get your protein and fullness from foods like beans, lentils and squash. Add grains like brown, black or wild rice. You can also try grains like quinoa, millet, amaranth, and barley. Find these grains and rice at any health food stores and at some neighborhood stores (depending on the neighborhood). Find various recipes on the internet or ask your friends and neighbors about dishes that they prepared with certain veggies.

You'll be surprised at just how easy, fun, creative, and filling it can be to create meals without animal products. You may also be surprised at how good you feel when you do!

10. Taste the Rainbow: When you are preparing your foods, try to choose varieties of the more common foods that are different colors from what you normally get. Of course, I'm speaking of produce and not items that have a different combination of food colorings! Instead of always eating green bell peppers, white rice, red beets, yellow onions, white cabbage, orange carrots, and red tomatoes, try to have red/yellow/orange bell peppers, black rice, golden beets, red onions, purple cabbage, white or purple carrots, and yellow tomatoes. This will allow you the familiarity of that particular food while still allowing you to go outside of your comfort zone and try something new. Then, begin to buy colorful produce that you know about but rarely eat. Pick up some blueberries, blackberries, or mangoes. Try red leaf lettuce instead of iceberg lettuce. Have purple and green kale or even yellow and white chard instead of spinach.

11. Read the Labels: Learning to read labels can be a crucial part of gaining/regaining control of your health. The more you know what to look for and how to decipher the marketing codes on boxes and packages, the better you will be at making better choices for you and your family.

12. Load up on Fiber: Fiber acts like the broom that sweeps your body clean. The more fiber you have in your diet, the more you decrease constipation, cholesterol, various cancers (including colon), diverticulosis, gallstone formation, and a myriad of other maladies. Fiber rich foods help you feel fuller for longer, which can help you decrease or stop snacking. This can help you get to and maintain a healthy weight. Refer back to Chapter 6, "Empty Your Trash!" for ideas on ways to add more fiber rich foods in your diet.

13. Experiment!! There are some recipes in the back of this book that you can try out. Use them. Incorporate them into your meals. Once you do that, make changes to them. Make them

easier and more palatable to you. Make it your own. Don't be afraid of doing something that you have never done before.

14. Get the family involved: Let members of your family, especially children, pick a recipe to be prepared for the next meal. Let them help purchase, prepare, and present the dish. The more involved they are in the process, the more likely that they will participate.

15. Pick A New One: Go to a store in a different neighborhood and check out the selection of fruit, veggies and meats. Pick one that you are not familiar with and try it out. Find a few recipes, to prepare this food so that you can have multiple experiences with it. Don't decide that you don't like something until you've tried it several different ways. You may not like it raw, but you may like it sautéed or in a casserole or in a soup. Broaden your culinary horizons!

16. Go Organic: Buying organic food means that you are purchasing food that is not genetically modified (also known as GMO) and is not grown with any pesticides, herbicides, or other chemicals that can potentially harm you. In your journey to health, you want to decrease the amount of chemicals you put in your body so that you body has less to clear out later. This decreases the burden placed on the organs of elimination and frees up energy that your body can use to heal and grow the way you want it to. I do realize that purchasing all organic foods can put a bit of a strain on the wallet for some people, so to help with that try focusing on the "Dirty Dozen" list. This is a list that the Environmental Working Group puts together each year to let us know the 12 produce crops that are the MOST heavily sprayed. By purchasing these 12 organic, even if nothing else is organic, we can get rid of about 75% of the chemicals that we would normally ingest from our foods. Isn't that AMAZING??!! So, check out Appendix B for that list. Take the list with you when you go shopping so that you can be aware of what to buy organic.

"What you eat becomes a part of you"
– Dr. Ayesha Worsham

I think it's important for me to say (or repeat) that by no means am I saying that changing your eating habits will clear away all your health problems and you'll never get sick. Of course, it's possible that you may never get sick again, but I cannot make that guarantee. What I can promise is that eating better will set you up to be much less likely to get ill and much more likely to heal and have boundless energy!!

CHAPTER 13

Let's Eat!

ℭ ✠ ℬↄ

And when you crush an apple with your teeth, say to it in your heart, "Your seeds shall live in my body and the buds of your tomorrow Shall blossom in my heart, and your fragrance shall be my breath, And together we shall rejoice through all the seasons."
– Kahlil Gibran, *The Prophet*

Here is the fun part! It's time to eat. In this section I present to you recipes that will help you eat better. Most of those recipes will be simple, clean, and healthful but there will be an occasional recipe that will be more complex. The more involved recipes will be for those that are feeling a bit braver.

Before we get into the recipes, I do want to bring up two points:

You must unlearn what you have learned - Yoda

1. There is no such thing as breakfast, lunch, and dinner food. Food is food. Food is Fuel. Eat what is going to nourish your body. Eat what is going to give you the most fuel, nutrients, and building blocks for your cells. Get out of the mindset of breakfast foods that must be carb-filled, sugary dish that will give you an energy crash at midmorning. No bueno!
2. Don't over-shop. It's much better to purchase food for the week and eat all the food you purchase than it is to purchase food for the month and throw away a bunch of it. In essence, you are wasting money on food that goes bad. That was your

hard earned money that could have been used on better quality food instead of being thrown away. Fresher is better. You are saving more money because you aren't over-shopping and your food is fresher & tastier.

I've chosen recipes that I have personally used and some that I've given to patients that I've been treated. I will share with you where I got these recipes in case you'd like to go and explore the resources further for more recipes to use and experiment with. Most of these recipes will be vegetarian and vegan. Of course you can make substitutions as you would like, but I'd suggest that you try to eat as many plant based foods as possible to help improve the quality of your health.

I also got recipes from my very good friend, Dr. Ayesha Worsham. She is a true health food foodie. She is the consummate "*Flexitarian*" in that her meals range from Vegan, Raw Foodist to Regular meat-n-potatoes type meals. All of which are clean, healthy and extremely delicious. It's because of her that I've grown to love many of the food choices that I eat today.

Ok, now that that's been said, look through the different sections of this chapter and experiment. Try stuff. Live a little. Make it fun and enjoy yourself!! **Bon Appetite** and **Laissez Les Bon Temps Rouler**!

Some of the recipes below were obtained from the resources noted:
i.   Raw Foods for Busy People by Jordan Maerin
ii. The Raw Truth: The Recipe for Reversing Diabetes by Kirt Tyson, NMD
iii. The Juicing Bible by Pat Crocker
iv. Vegan Soul Kitchen by Bryant Terry
v.   Dr. Ayesha Worsham

SPA WATER
This is the type of water that you would find in those high end spas to be served to their patrons as a refreshing drink. The following recipes are GREAT ways to incorporate more water into your day in a healthy,

colorful, tasty way that you and your family will LOVE! Try these, and then get innovative! Create new combinations daily. Try new blends based on color, taste, season, or just what you have available.

For each of these water recipes slice the fruit or veggies as thinly as possible and put them in the container. If you are adding mint or other herbs, slightly bruise it to help release the flavor. Add ice if desired. Then fill the container with Filtered, Reverse Osmoses, Spring Water or even Sparkling Mineral Water for a twist. Use more or less fruit/veggies depending on how lightly or intensely flavored you want your water to be. Put it in beautiful container and set it in the refrigerator to chill. Drink throughout the day.

Cucumber Citrus Water

> 1 cucumber
> 1 lemon
> 1-2 oranges
> 2 limes
> 1 bunch of mint

-can divide into four 24 ounce bottles, three 1 liter containers, or a gallon.

Blueberry Mint Water

> 2 cup blueberries
> 2 sprigs of mint

Strawberry Basil Water

> 10 strawberries
> 3 basil leaves

Citrus Water

> 1 orange
> 1 lime
> ½ lemon
> 1 grapefruit

Berry Blast

 10 strawberries

 2 cups blueberries

Spicy Lemon Refresher

 1 lemon

 3 inch peeled ginger root

Ginger Mint Water

 1 knob ginger, thinly sliced and bruised

 3 sprigs fresh mint, rosemary, or basil slightly bruised

Cucumber Rosemary Cooler

 10 slices cucumber

 1 sprig fresh rosemary

Cucumber Citrus Mint Refresher

 12 slices cucumber

 4 slices lemon

 4 sprigs fresh mint

 2 sprigs fresh rosemary

OTHER BEVERAGES

Homemade Brown Rice Milk – *If you are looking for a dairy milk alternative, but thought that alternate milks were a bit expensive in the stores, this is an inexpensive, easy alternative that you may want to consider. Easy to make and tasty to drink!* This recipe was taken from the http://happyherbivore.com/2011/08/what-is-rice-milk-rice-milk-recipe/

 1/3 cup uncooked rice

 1 tsp. vanilla extract

 Sweetener to taste, (ex: maple syrup, stevia, agave, molasses, date sugar, etc.)

-Bring 1 cup of water to a boil. Add rice and bring to a boil again. Once boiling, cover, reduce heat to low, and simmer until rice is cooked, about 40 minutes. The rice will be soft and waterlogged. Drain off any excess water if necessary. Transfer rice to a blender and add 2 cups of warm water. Blend until well incorporated, about 2-3 minutes. Add another cup of warm water and blend again. If you prefer thinner, add warm water, ½ to 1 cup at a time and blend again. Let the mixture sit for 30 minutes. Scoop away any residue off the top of your milk mixture. Once removed, slowly pour the milk into a container through a strainer or cheesecloth. Squeeze or press the rest of the milk out of the solid matter. Add a few drops of vanilla extract and/or sweetener to taste.

Homemade Nut Milk – makes 2 servings
Making your own nut milk can be a fun and rewarding experience. It can save you money and you can taste the freshness of the beverage. On top of that, you know exactly what's in it! You can use any variety of nuts that you want to experience. Your choices can be a single nut or seed (almond, hazelnut, Brazil nut, cashew, hemp seeds, sunflower seeds, etc.) or a combination. This milk can be used in smoothies, shakes, soups, cereals, or any recipe that calls for milk. You can even drink it as a stand-alone beverage. Again, be creative and experiment.

> 1 cup raw almonds soaked in water overnight in the refrigerator and drained
> 3 cups filtered water
> 1 tsp. vanilla or almond extract (optional)
> 1 tsp. ground cinnamon (optional)
> 2-3 pitted dates OR ½ tsp. maple syrup OR ½ tsp. other natural sweetener to taste (optional)

-Drain and discard the water from the soaked almonds. Add the 3 cups of water, almonds and dates to a blender and blend until almost smooth. Add ½ cup more water for a thinner consistency if desired. Strain the blended mixture using cheesecloth or some other strainer. Milk will keep well in the refrigerator for up to 4 days.

Easy Root Coffee (iii)

The recipe is a great alternative to regular (instant) coffee with the added benefit of being cleansing and supportive to the liver, kidneys, and adrenal glands. Mix it like 'instant' coffee.

> ½ cup powdered chicory root
> ¼ cup powdered dandelion root
> ¼ cup powdered burdock root
> ¼ cup powdered carob
> 1 tbsp. ground ginseng

-In a mixing bowl, combine all the ingredients. Transfer to an airtight jar to store.

-To make 1 cup, measure 1 tbsp. root blend into a mug and pour boiling water over. Stir and allow solids to settle on the bottom (or strain) before drinking.

Raspberry Tea (iii) - *"This tea calms the muscles and nerves"*

> ¼ cup raspberries, fresh or frozen
> 1 tsp. raspberry leaves
> 1 tsp. lemon balm
> 2 cups boiling water

-Combine ingredients in a non-reactive container. Cover with boiling water and steep for 15 minutes. Strain into cups and drink warm.

Lavender Tea (iii) - *"This antioxidant tea stimulates circulation and digestion. It is also relaxing and liver supportive."*

> 2 parts lemon balm
> 1 part lavender flowers
> 1 part German chamomile flowers
> 1 part passionflower

-combine ingredients into an airtight container and store in a cool, dark, dry place.

-To make tea, measure 1 tsp. blend per 1 cup water. Put tea blend into a non-reactive container. Pour boiling water into container. Cover and steep for 15 minutes. Strain into cups. Relax and enjoy!

-NOTE: a 'part' can be any amount of measurement you want it to be (pinch, tsp., cup, gallon, etc.). Just remember to be consistent with each.

SMOOTHIES

These various smoothie recipes can act as a meal replacement, protein shake, or help you get your daily fruit and veggies in. Try different combinations. Don't just try the fruit varieties, but also try those with veggies. You'll find that you can appreciate those as well. These are also great ways to introduce more veggies into your children's diets without as much hassle and fighting.

For all the smoothie recipes, place all ingredients in a blender and blend until desired consistency. Add more or less fluid to give desired thickness. You may need to tamp the foods down the sides of your blender occasionally in order to make sure that you get the best mixture. It also may help if you put the lighter items (etc.: leaves) in the blender first before adding heavier items (etc.: frozen fruit). This can help you get the best blend with the least amount of effort. The better quality your blender, the better blended your smoothies will be. This will make them taste better overall. Use what you have until you have the opportunity to upgrade equipment. As always, the last ingredient is always ENJOY YOURSELF!!

NOTE: If you want a really, really creamy smoothie without adding milk and yogurt or adding the sweetness and carbs of a banana, then add an AVOCADO! It will make all your smoothies very smooth and creamy and it won't alter the flavor (though it may alter the color a bit depending on how much avocado you use and the color of your other ingredients). As an added bonus, you'll get all the terrific, healing oils, proteins, and nutrients that make the avocado such a wonderful, beautifying fruit. TRUST ME! You'll LOVE it!

Glowing Green Smoothie – *This is the cornerstone recipe for Kimberly Snyder's Beauty Detox Solution*

  1 ½ cups water

  1 head organic romaine lettuce, chopped

  ½ head of large bunch or ¾ of small bunch organic spinach

  3-4 stalks organic celery

  1 organic apple, cored and chopped

  1 organic pear, cored and chopped

  1 organic banana

  Juice of ½ organic lemon

  1/3 bunch organic cilantro, stems okay (optional)

  1/3 bunch organic parsley, stems okay (optional)

-Add water and chopped head of romaine and spinach to the blender. Starting the blender on a low speed, mix until smooth. Gradually moving to higher speeds, add the celery, apple and pear. Add the cilantro and parsley if you choose. Add the banana and lemon juice last

Oatmeal Breakfast Smoothie

  1 Ripe Banana

  ½ Cup Frozen Pineapple Chunks

  ¼ Cup Oats, Rolled

  ½ Cup Almond Milk

  2 tsps. Flaxseeds

  2 tsps. Agave Nectar or Pure Maple Syrup

-Place all ingredients into a blender and mix to desired consistency. Add milk/water as needed

Cherry Anti-inflammatory Smoothie

  ½ cup coconut flesh – fresh or frozen

  ½ cup frozen cherries

  5-8 fresh basil leaves

  1-2 cups coconut water or plain water

  1 tbsp. chia or hemp seeds

'Caramel' Apple Shake (i)

- 1 apple, cut in chunks
- 1 cup apple juice
- 2-3 tbsp. almond butter
- 2 tbsp. maple syrup OR 3 pitted soft dates
- Dash of cinnamon and nutmeg
- 1 ripe banana (optional)

Apple, Ginger, Avocado Pudding (v)

- 1 avocado
- 2-3 medium apples, peeled, cored, and cut
- 1 chunk fresh ginger
- 1-2 tsp. lemon juice (optional)

Calming Chamomile Smoothie (iii) – *great calming recipe*

- ½ cup soymilk or nut milk
- 1 apple, peeled, cored and chunked
- ¼ cantaloupe, cut into chunks
- 2 tbsp. yogurt, coconut or soy work very well
- 1 tbsp. fresh German chamomile flowers or 1 tsp. dried leaves
- 1 tbsp. sesame seeds (optional) to thicken this drink

Avocado Pineapple Smoothie (iii)

- 1 cup pineapple chunks, fresh or frozen
- ¾ cup raspberry juice
- 1 avocado, pitted

JUICES

In order to make juices, wash all produce well then run all ingredients through a juicer, putting a small amount of produce in at a time. Ideally you want to drink the juice within about 15 minutes of making it, to ensure the full preservation of its enzymes and all its nutrients. If you can't drink it right away, cover it in an airtight container and keep it cold. Drink it within a few hours. Don't just gulp your juice down though. "Chew your juice" by allowing it to stay in your mouth for a few moments so that the enzymes in your mouth can begin to break the larger molecules down and make it easier for your body to absorb nutrients.

Also keep in mind that any of the leafy greens can be switched out. Try a variety in your juices. You can try what's available, what's in season, or what you happen to have in your fridge. Play around and get creative!

Glowing Green Juice – *Kimberly Snyder's signature juice in The Beauty Detox Solution*
     1 bunch organic kale or 1 bunch organic spinach
     3-4 stalks organic celery
     1 small organic apple, cut in quarters
     Juice of ½ an organic lemon

Mean Green Juice – *This is the juice made famous by Joe Cross in the movie 'Fat, Sick, and Nearly Dead.' If you've never seen the movie, I'd recommend that you go out and rent it (or watch it on Hulu for free!!) It could change your life!*
     1 cucumber
     4 celery stalks
     2 apples
     6-8 leaves of kale
     ½ lemon
     1 tbsp. ginger

Morning Green Glory Juice – *Another one of Joe Crosses' favorites, especially for breakfast. Try it in place of your morning coffee. You won't believe how much energy you can get! The perfect way to start your day. Your body will thank you for it.*
     4-5 large kale leaves
     1 large handful of spinach
     3 romaine leaves
     1 cucumber

3 celery stalks

1 green apple

1 lemon, peeled (You can leave the peel on but it will taste very bitter/tart. Might be overpowering. Try a small piece first.)

Crisp and Clean Green Juice – *Joe Crosses' Liver cleansing, anti-nausea, get-over-a-celebration juice.*

1 large wedge green cabbage

2 small pears

1 bunch romaine leaves

1" ginger root

Kale Lemonade

1 apple

1 bunch kale

½ lemon

1" knob ginger (optional) for a spicy kick

-You can hand squeeze the juice from the lemon or run the whole thing through the juicer (this will make it more potent and slightly bitter).

Carrot Cake Juice – *A Joe Cross, Team Reboot recipe*

4-6 large carrots

1 ½ sweet potatoes

1-2 red apple

Dash of cinnamon

Calming Chamomile Juice (iii)

2 apples

1 stalk celery

¼ cup chamomile tea

-Make a pot of chamomile tea. Process apples and celery through a juicer. Add in tea. Mix. Drink.

FRUIT SALADS
Nutty, Fruity, Protein Salad (v)

1 Mango, cut into chunks

1 Large Avocado, Cut into slices

2 tbsp. raw Sesame Seeds

2 tbsp. Lime Juice

-Mix ingredients in a bowl. Eat half, save the other half for later.

Mango, Blackberry Salad (v)

1 Mango, cut into chunks

1 pint Blackberries

-Mix ingredients in a bowl. Eat half, save the other half for later

Red, Green, and Black Salad (v)

1 handful blackberries or blueberries

½ Cup Honey Dew Melon

1 handful of Strawberries, sliced

-Mix ingredients in a bowl. Eat while smiling

Cinnamon Stewed Fruit, Raw (i) – *No cooking needed. Delicious and full of nutrients!*

4 ripe apples, pears, or peaches, sliced

2 tbsp. lemon juice

1 tsp. lemon zest

½ cup apple juice

1 tbsp. cinnamon or pumpkin pie spice

1 tbsp. agave or maple syrup (optional)

½ cup raisins or currants (optional)

¼ cup chopped or ground pecans or nuts (optional)

-Toss all ingredients and let it to marinate for at least an hour, allowing the lemon juice to soften fruit

VEGETABLE SALADS

Root Salad (v)

Grate 1 small beet, 1 small kohlrabi, and 1 carrot.

-Sprinkle lemon or lime juice. Toss. Eat.

<u>Mustard Green Salad</u> (v)

      Mustard Greens, Gut into small pieces

      EVOO

      Lemon Juice

      Salt

      Sunflower Seed

-Cut Greens. Sprinkle in lemon juice and massage greens for 1 minute. Add EVOO, Salt and Seeds. Toss. Eat. Remember to chew well. The more you chew, the more peppery it gets.

<u>Probiotic & Enzyme Salad</u>

This recipe is taken from <u>The Beauty Detox Solution</u>. This is a great version of Sauerkraut. The healthy bacteria combined with the health benefits of the cabbage and ginger are a super combination.

Four 24 ounce or three 32 ounce clean glass jars that have been sterilized by dipping them in boiled water

      1 medium head of green (or purple) cabbage, shredded or finely sliced by hand

      Leave 6 of the large outer leaves to the side, intact

      4 cups water

      4 inches gingerroot, peeled and grated

      1 tbsp. unpasteurized miso paste

-Place the shredded cabbage in a large mixing bowl. Blend the water, ginger and miso in blender until smooth. Pour mixture over the shredded cabbage. Mix very well. Pack the mixture into sterilized jars glass jars. Use a wooden spoon to really pack the mixture tightly. Leave 2 inches of room at the top of the jars so the salad has room to expand. Fold a few of the outer cabbage leaves into very tight rolls, and place them on top of the mixture to fill that 2-inch space. Tightly close jars. Leave the jars in your pantry for 5 days. Be sure the room temperature is around 65 and 70 degrees. If slightly colder, wrap a towel around each jar and keep in the pantry. After the 5 days, remove the outer cabbage leaves and discard. Move the jars to the refrigerator (which slows down the fermentation process). Bubbling is a good sign that healthy probiotics are teeming. Enjoy at least ½ cup at dinner every night, and also at lunch, when possible. Once the seal has been broken on each jar, the salad will keep in the refrigerator for up to 1 month.

CONDIMENTS, DIPS SAUCES, AND DRESSINGS

Store all condiments, dips and dressings in the refrigerator when not in use. Because they are fresh dressings with no preservatives, they will probably only keep for a week or two so be sure to use them all up after you make them. With tastes this fantastic, I'm sure that won't be a problem!

Avocado Dressing – *this is a truly creamy, delicious dressing that adds a powerful nutrient punch of essential oils and other nutrients to every salad or used in place of mayonnaise. I got the idea when I had an avocado dressing at a restaurant. I didn't know what was in theirs so I tried to recreate it on my own. Not bad if I do say so myself!*

    2 ripe avocadoes

    3 tbsp. lemon juice

    1-2 cloves garlic (to taste)

    ¼ cup red onions or scallions

    1 tbsp. seasoning of your choice (Italian seasoning, salt/pepper, dried dill, rosemary, etc.)

    ¼ cup coconut milk

-Blend all ingredients together. Add water or coconut milk to desired consistency.

-Alternate: add 1 ripe tomato to make an avocado tomato dressing

Ranch Dressing (i) – *this will only take about 2 minutes to make. You can't go wrong with that!*

    1 cup cashew butter

    ½ cup water or ¼ cup water + ¼ coconut milk

    3 tbsp. lemon juice

1 tsp. raw apple cider vinegar

1 tsp. Italian seasoning or dill

1-2 cloves garlic

1 celery stalk

-Blend until smooth and creamy

-Alternately, you can use celery salt instead of the celery stalk and salt.

Vinaigrette Dressing (i)– *This recipe can be used as a tasty marinade as well*

1 cup EVOO

½ cup raw apple cider vinegar or balsamic vinegar or a mixture of the two

2 cloves minced garlic or ½ tsp. garlic powder

2 tbsp. raw, local honey

1 tsp. salt and pepper

2 tsp. dried oregano

2 tsp. basil

Dried chili peppers to taste (for a spicy kick)

-Place in a jar to store. Shake well before each use.

-Alternately, for a Creamy Vinaigrette add 3-4 stalks of celery to the recipe

-Add 1-2 tbsp. Dijon mustard for a tangy twist

Raspberry Vinaigrette Dressing (i)

½ Vinaigrette Dressing from above

1 pint fresh or frozen raspberries

½ cup orange juice

1 chopped scallion

Pineapple Barbecue Sauce (i)

1 cup chopped fresh tomatoes

½ cup sun-dried tomatoes, soaked 15 minutes and chopped

2 tbsp. pineapple juice, plus ¼ cup pineapple chunks

¼ cup chopped onion

1 small clove garlic or 1/8 tsp. garlic powder

¼ tsp. cayenne or minced hot peppers

2 tbsp. maple syrup or to taste

2 tbsp. EVOO or sesame oil

1 tsp. salt or to taste

¼ tsp. each paprika and black pepper

-Combine all ingredients and blend until smooth

Creamy Pineapple Sauce (i) – *great to use as a fruit dip or as a sweet dressing on your salads*

¼ cup cashew or macadamia butter

¼ cup pineapple juice

1 tbsp. lemon juice

½ tbsp. EVOO

2 tsp. dried dill

-Whisk or blend ingredients together. If whisking, make sure nut butter is at room temperature. If blending, add dill last and gently pulse blend.

Instant Cinnamon Fruit Dip (i) – *Great dip to serve with sliced fruit.*

½ cup cashew or macadamia butter or tahini

½ cup orange juice or water

¼ cup honey or ½ cup soft dates

1 tsp. vanilla extract

1 tbsp. cinnamon or pumpkin spice

½ tsp. orange zest

-Blend nut butter with orange juice or water until smooth and creamy. Add honey or the dates (two at a time) and then add the rest of the ingredients. Add more juice or water until dip reaches desired consistency

Very Berry Fruit Dip (i)

1 ripe banana

½ ripe avocado

1 ½ cups fresh or frozen mixed berries

1-2 tbsp. lemon or orange juice

1-2 tsp. lemon or orange zest

1 tbsp. honey or maple syrup or ½ tbsp. date sugar
Chopped fresh mint or a pinch of dried mint
Pinch of sea salt
-Blend all ingredients until smooth and creamy

Mustard, Raw Vegan (ii)

½ cup mustard seeds
1 tsp. turmeric
¾ cup apple cider vinegar
1/3 cup water
½ tsp. lemon juice
¼ tsp. sea salt

-Grind mustard seeds. Place all ingredients in a blender. Store and refrigerate in a glass jar.

Ketchup, Raw Vegan (ii)

2 medium tomatoes
1 cup sun dried tomatoes
¼ cup apple cider vinegar
2 tbsp. yacon syrup (can try maple syrup or molasses instead) or
¼ cup soaked dates
1 tbsp. Nama Shoyu (raw soy sauce) or Braggs Liquid Aminos
2 cloves garlic

-Place all ingredients in a blender. Blend well. Serve immediately or dehydrate at 115o for 3 hours. Store in glass jar and refrigerate.

Fresh Plum Ketchup (iv)

1 tbsp. EVOO
½ cup diced red onion
½ cup diced red bell pepper
¼ tsp. paprika
2 cloves garlic, minced
1 8-ounce can chopped tomatoes
½ tsp. agave nectar
1 tbsp. red wine vinegar

2 tsp. tamari

3 ripe plums, peeled, pitted, and chopped

3 tbsp. freshly squeezed lemon juice

Course sea salt

Freshly ground white pepper

-In a large sauté pan over medium heat, combine EVOO, onion, bell pepper and paprika. Sauté for 8-10 minutes, stirring often, until the vegetables begin to caramelize. Add the garlic and sauté until fragrant, about 2 minutes. Add the tomatoes, agave, vinegar, and tamari. Reduce the heat to low, cover, and simmer, stirring occasionally, until thickening, about 15 minutes. Remove from the heat. Stir in the plums and lemon juice and set aside to cool. Transfer the ketchup to an upright blender and puree until smooth. Season with salt and pepper to taste. Store in an airtight container in the refrigerator for up to a week.

Mayonnaise, Raw Vegan (ii)

2 cups macadamia nuts

1 ½ cups water

2 cloves garlic

½ cup lemon juice

1 tbsp. apple cider vinegar

½ tsp. sea salt

½ tsp. stone ground mustard

-Combine all ingredients in a blender except water. Blend and add water to reach a creamy texture. Store and refrigerate in a glass jar.

Mayonnaise, Raw Vegan – from *Liquid Raw: The Complete Book of Raw Food*

1 cup raw cashews

2 young Thai coconuts (meat only)

½ cup pure water

1 tsp. Celtic sea salt

1/8 tsp. cayenne

1 tsp. raw honey or light agave

1 lemon (juice only)

½ cup or more cold-pressed EVOO

-Combine all the ingredients (except the oil) together in a high speed blender and blend. Add oil slowly.

Alkaline Guacamole by Health-e-Solutions (modified)

    1 avocado, smashed

    1 tbsp. red onion, diced

    3 tbsp. julienne cut sun dried tomatoes

    ½ tsp. fresh lemon juice (to taste)

    Salt and Pepper (to taste)

-Mix all ingredients in a small bowl. Use as a spread on bread, sandwiches, on salads, or as a dip on slice veggies.

Avocado Pasta Sauce

This is a great, no-cook pasta sauce that you can use for a creamy, meat-less (or add meat if you'd like) pasta dish. It is especially good to use on Spaghetti Squash as a vegan, tasty, 'low-carb' pasta meal! This recipe can be seen on http://ohsheglows.com/2011/01/31/15-minute-creamy-avocado-pasta/

    1 medium avocado, pitted

    ½ lemon, juiced + lemon zest to garnish

    1-3 garlic cloves, to taste

    ½ tsp. Kosher salt, to taste

    ¼ cup fresh basil (optional)

    2 tbsp. EVOO

    2 servings / 6 ounces of pasta (try spaghetti squash recipe in "entrée" section)

    Freshly ground black pepper, to taste

-Place garlic cloves, lemon juice and EVOO into a blender or food processor. Blend until smooth. Add avocado, basil, and salt. Process until smooth and creamy. Pour sauce on pasta and toss until fully combined. Garnish with lemon zest and black pepper. Serve immediately. Makes 2 servings.

ENTREES AND SIDES

Brown Coconut Rice (iv)

I was first introduced to coconut rice in Belize. It was an experience that I'll never forget! A simple twist to a regular dish that was rich and flavorful. It was eaten with every dish. It was most memorable with fresh caught fish and veggies. Deeeeee-lish!

> 1 cup short-grain rice
>
> ¾ cup coconut milk
>
> 1 ½ cup water
>
> ½ tsp. Course sea salt
>
> 3 tbsp. unsweetened shredded coconut (optional)

-Add ingredients to a medium sized saucepan over medium heat and bring to a boil. Reduce heat to low, cover and simmer until all liquid evaporates, about 40-45 minutes. Remove from heat and keep covered for 10 more minutes. Fluff with a fork. Serve. ENJOY!

Baked BBQ Black-Eyed Peas (iv) *—modified from original recipe. This recipe is more detailed, but it's worth it! You'll definitely enjoy it!*

> 1 ½ cups dried black-eyed peas, soaked overnight, drained and rinsed (or use canned for beginners)
>
> 3 tbsp. plus 2 tsp. EVOO
>
> ½ cup diced green bell pepper
>
> 2 tbsp. red wine vinegar
>
> 2 tbsp. freshly squeezed lime juice
>
> ½ cup tamari or low sodium soy sauce
>
> 1 cup canned tomato sauce
>
> 1 large chipotle chili in adobo sauce
>
> ¼ cup agave nectar or maple syrup
>
> 1 tbsp. ground cumin
>
> Pinch of cayenne
>
> 1 tsp. dried thyme

-If using dried beans, add to medium size sauce pan with just enough water to cover them and ring to a boil. Reduce heat to medium-low and cook until tender, 50-60 minutes. Drain beans are reserve water.

-While beans are cooking, combine 2 tsp. EVOO, the onions, and bell pepper in a medium-sized sauté pan over medium heat. Sauté for 5-7 minutes, or until the vegetables soften. Add the garlic and cook for another 2 minutes, until fragrant.

-Preheat the oven to 350°F

-BBQ Sauce: In a blender, combine the vinegar, lime juice, tamari, tomato sauce, chili, agave, cumin, cayenne, thyme, 1 cup of reserved bean water, and the remaining EVOO. Puree for 30 seconds until smooth.

-In a cast-iron skillet or a 2-quart baking dish, combine the cooked beans with the sautéed vegetables, and BBQ sauce and stir well. Bake, uncovered, for 2 hours, stirring occasionally. Serve at room temp.

Mashed Cauliflower – Cooked

This recipe is a GREAT alternative to mashed potatoes when trying to decrease caloric intake and increase veggies!!

  1 Medium Head of Cauliflower

  1 tbsp. Extra Virgin Olive Oil (EVOO)

  1/8 tsp. freshly ground black pepper – to taste

  Sea Salt – to taste

  ½ tsp. chopped fresh or dry chives for garnish

  ½ tsp. minced garlic (optional)

  ¼ Cup vegan Grated Parmesan (optional)

  1/8 tsp. chicken base or vegan Bullion (optional)

  3 tbsp. Earth Balance or unsalted vegan butter (optional)

-Bring a large pot of salted water to boil. Add cauliflower florets and cook until very tender. This will take about 8-10 minutes. Save ¼ cup of the cooking water and drain the rest. Pat Cauliflower dry with a paper towel. Place cooked cauliflower in food processer or blender and add oil, reserved water a little bit at a time, until smooth. Alternately, you can mash the cauliflower with a potato masher. Season with salt and pepper. Use other seasonings as desired. Garnish with Chives. Serve warm.

<u>Mashed Cauliflower – raw</u> (from www.ChoosingRaw.com/Steak-And-Potatoes/)

> 2 ½ cups raw cashews or macadamias or pine nuts (soaked in water for 30 minutes for best results)
> 1 tsp. sea salt
> 2 tbsp. mellow white miso
> 3 tbsp. lemon juice (to taste)
> 1 tbsp. EVOO
> Pepper to taste
> 4 cups cauliflower, chopped into small florets and pieces
> 1/3 cup (or less) water

-Place cashews and salt in a food processor, and process into a fine powder. Next, add miso, lemon juice, pepper and cauliflower. Pulse to combine. With the motor of the machine running, add water in a thin stream until the mixture takes on a smooth, whipped texture. Stop frequently to clean the sides of the bowl if necessary. 6 servings

-Alternately, use raw, unsalted cashew nut butter instead of whole nuts

-For diabetics, cashews are not the best choice. Instead, try half macadamia nuts and pine nuts.

-Can also add garlic, rosemary, or Italian seasoning for a variation on flavor

<u>Meatless, Marinated Steak</u> – (from www.ChoosingRaw.com/steak-and-potatoes/)

"Meat":

> 4 Portobello mushroom caps

Marinade:

> 1/3 cup EVOO
> ¼ cup balsamic vinegar
> ¼ cup maple syrup
> 3 tbsp. nama shoyu (raw soy sauce) or regular soy sauce
> Sprinkle pepper

-Submerge 4 Portobello caps in marinade. Let them stay in marinade 1 hour at minimum, though overnight in the fridge is even better.

Eggplant "Parmesan" by Health-e-Solutions
This recipe has three parts, Eggplant "Parmesan" (no cheese included), Parmesan, and marinara sauce. I've made this a few times. Trust me…. You'll love it!

A. Eggplant "Parmesan":
     3 large eggplants
     Grape seed oil
     2 cups almond meal
     2 cups flaxseed meal
     1 tsp. salt
     ½ tsp. pepper

B. "Parmesan" mixture:
-Mix the almond meal, flaxseed meal, salt and pepper in a small bowl
-Variations: you can add different spices like basil or oregano

C. Marinara Sauce:
     1 brown onion diced
     1 clove garlic crushed
     2 tbsp. grape seed oil
     8 large tomatoes chopped finely
     1 tsp. basil
     1 tsp. oregano
     1 tsp. salt
     ½ tsp. pepper
-Place grape seed oil in sauce pan. On low heat, sauté onion until just tender. Turn off heat and take pan off burner. Stir in crushed garlic. Stir combination for about 1 minute. Place chopped tomatoes, basil, oregano, salt and pepper in pan. Stir thoroughly.
-For Meal: Preheat oven to 400°. Cut eggplant into ½ inch slices. Make "parmesan" mixture. Lightly grease baking sheet with grape seed oil.

Taking an eggplant slice, first dip the slice in a bowl and coat both sides with oil. Then dip the slice in the "parmesan" mixture. Coat the slice generously. Then place the slice on the greased baking sheet. Repeat this process until all slices are prepared. Bake in preheated oven for 20 minutes. Turn slices over and bake another 20 minutes or until tender. Remove from oven and spread a light coat of Marina sauce over each eggplant slice. You can sprinkle a little extra parmesan mixture over the Marinara sauce as a garnish.

Roasted Spaghetti Squash

Spaghetti squash has a stringy texture when cooked, making it an ideal replacement for regular pasta. It is non-processed (because you're using whole squash) and it's a veggie. This can boost your daily veggie and fiber intake when eaten with a hearty, chunky sauce.

> 1 Spaghetti Squash
> 1 tsp. EVOO
> Sea Salt and Black Pepper to taste

-Preheat oven to 375oF. Slice down the middle lengthwise. You may need to use a rocking motion to cut through it. With a metal ice cream scoop or spoon, scoop out the seeds and guts. Set aside the seeds if you want to roast them later. Brush halves with tiny amount of EVOO (about ½ tsp. each side). Sprinkle with freshly ground black pepper, sea salt, or any seasoning you'd like. Place on a baking sheet lined with parchment paper, cut sound down. Roast at 375F for about 35-45 minutes or until you can easily scrape strands away from the squash (time will vary depending on size of squash). The outer yellow skin will also deepen in color. Remove from oven and flip each half. If it's ready (use a fork to see if you can scrape strands easily) allow it to cool for 5-10 minutes. Once cooled, grab a fork and scrape the flesh over and over WITH the grain of the squash. You'll be left with a bunch of spaghetti-like strands! Season again. Add sauce if using. Serve immediately.
-This can be paired with any spaghetti sauce, marinara sauce (try it with the recipe above), pesto, chili, stew, or the creamy avocado pasta sauce (found in the "sauces" section above).

SOUPS AND BROTHS

When you make your fresh vegetable juices or when you slice your vegetables for your meals, put them in Ziplocs bags and store them in the freezer for later. You can even use the tough stems and trimmings from your leafy greens. Use them in your stocks, broths and soups. This way you never create waste! You can even make your stocks in batches and freeze it in ice trays for easy use in small or large dishes. Stock will keep in refrigerator for up to 2 days.

Vegetable Broth Stock

      1 tbsp. EVOO

      2 large onions, including skin

      1-2 large carrot, sliced

      4 ribs celery including leaves, sliced

      1 bunch green onions, chopped

      8 ounces mushrooms, stems included

      1 whole bulb garlic, unpeeled and smashed with back of knife

      2 bay leaves

      1 tsp. dried parsley OR 8 sprigs fresh parsley

      1 tsp. dried thyme OR 3 sprigs fresh thyme

      ½ tsp. coarse sea salt

      1/8 tsp. cayenne

      9 cups water

-Chop veggies into 1 inch chunks. Heat oil in a soup pot. Add veggies and seasonings. Cook over high heat for 5-10 minutes, stirring frequently. Add salt and water and bring to a boil. Lower heat and simmer, uncovered, for 30 minutes. Strain. Discard veggies

-Other ingredients to consider include: eggplant, asparagus (butt ends), corn cobs, fennel (stalks and trimmings), bell peppers, pea pods, chard (stem and leaves), basil, potato skins... you get the idea.

Garlic Broth (iv)

      4 whole garlic bulbs, unpeeled, smashed with the back of a knife

      ½ tsp. sea salt

      9 cups water

-In a large pot over high heat, combine the ingredients and bring to a boil. Reduce heat to medium-low, and simmer uncovered for about 1 hour. Strain garlic cloves, pressing down on them to extract all liquid. Discard solids. Freeze whatever you won't use immediately.

Cream of Spinach Soup   http://www.chow.com/recipes/29216-vegan-cream-of-spinach-soup
The first time I tried this recipe, I... was... in.... LOVE!! Be sure to experiment with different veggies and different cream soups.

> 2 cups raw organic fresh spinach
> 1 cup organic zucchini (about 1 zucchini)
> 1 cup chopped red onions (about 1 medium onion)
> ¼ cup scallions or green onions (about 6)
> ¼ cup flat leaf parsley (a handful)
> 1 large stalk celery, chopped
> 4 cups strong vegetable broth
> 1 whole roasted garlic bulb
> ¼ - ½ cup raw cashews
> Dash of fresh lemon juice to taste
> Celtic sea salt to taste

-Place the garlic whole in the over on about 400 for about 30 minutes until soft and roasted
-In a saucepan, sauté onions and scallions with a pinch of Celtic sea salt to bring out the sweetness, until translucent. Add in spinach, celery, zucchini and parsley and cook for about 5 minutes. Add in stock and squeeze in roasted garlic pulp and bring to a boil. Simmer for about 20 minutes until veggies are cooked through. Allow to cool slightly and then puree in the blender with the cashews and return to the stove to warm and serve. Serve sprinkled with parsley.

Barley Soup
http://vegetarian.about.com/od/soupsstewsandchili/r/barleyvegetable.htm

> 1 onion, diced

2 cloves garlic, minced

8-9 cups water or vegetable broth

¾ cup barley, uncooked

2 carrots, diced

1 ½ cups cabbage, sliced

1 zucchini, sliced

1 24 ounce can diced or crushed tomatoes

2 bay leaves

¼ cup fresh parsley OR 1 tsp. Italian seasoning

Salt and pepper to taste

-In a large stock pot, sauté garlic and onions in olive oil for 4-5 minutes, until just barely soft. Carefully add broth and remaining ingredients and bring to a slow simmer. Allow to cook until barley is soft, about 30 minutes, preferably longer. Adjust seasonings as desired.

DESSERTS AND SNACKS

Peanut Butter and Dates I first heard about this combination from Chef Ahki. Since then, it's one of my go-to snacks. It's sooooooo good and simple!

> Fresh Dates
>
> Peanut Butter

-Dip the fresh dates in the peanut butter. Eat! Be sure to take the seeds out the dates before you bite done too hard on them.

-Option: try to get the natural, unsweetened peanut butter. You can also just go to a health food store and grind your own nuts into butter. Then you know it's fresh and there's nothing added.

-Alternative: try other nut butters like almond butter, hazelnut butter, tahini, and soy nut butter .

Cherry Cheesecake Bites (raw, vegan)
I haven't tried this recipe yet, but it looks simply DIVINE!!! And it only takes about 10-15 min. to make! I got this recipe from: http://www.ohbiteit.com/2012/06/cherry-cheesecake-bites.html

Fresh cherries or cherries in a jar

> 1 container or block of vegan cream cheese
>
> 1 cup powdered sugar
>
> Gram Cracker Crumbs – enough to cover cherries

-In a food processor or blender, combine cream cheese and powdered sugar. Once blended, add to a bowl. Put Gram Cracker crumbs in a separate bowl. Dip cherries in sweetened cream cheese then in the crumbs. Eat!

Avocado Based Pudding (i) – *This is one that you've GOT to try! Once I tried it, I was hooked. So very creamy and delicious. You'd never know that it was dairy-free!*

> 1 ripe avocado
>
> 1 ripe banana OR ¼ cup pitted dates, soaked 10 minutes
>
> ½ cup berries OR ¼ cup raw carob powder (if you want a chocolate pudding)
>
> 2 tsp. vanilla extract

-Blend all ingredients until smooth and creamy. Use spatula to scrape the sides of the container

Nut Based Pudding (i)

> 1 cup cashews soaked 30 minutes or almonds soaked 8 hours
>
> ½ cup water, orange juice or coconut water
>
> 1 ripe banana OR ¼ cup pitted dates, soaked in water 10 minutes
>
> ½ cup dried or fresh coconut (optional)
>
> Sliced banana or fresh berries of your choice

-Blend the nuts and water or juice first, until truly smooth, before adding the rest of the ingredients.

Berry Pops (iii) – *Makes 12 pops. This recipe reminds me of the* Frozen Cups *we used to eat when I was a child. ALWAYS a great summer time treat!*

> 2 cups raspberry, strawberry or cherry juice
>
> ½ cup freshly squeezed orange juice

½ cup beet juice

2 tbsp. liquid honey (optional)

-In a medium bowl, combine raspberry juice, orange juice, beet juice and honey. Pour ¼ cup juice into each waxed paper cup. Freeze for 1 hour or until firm enough to hold a stick. Insert wooden stick in middle and return to freezer for 1 hour or until hard.

Chocolate Chia Pudding – *from Liquid Raw*

¼ cup chia seeds

1 cup chocolate cashew milk or chocolate almond milk or chocolate coconut milk

½ tsp. alcohol-free vanilla extract

-Using a fork, mix all the ingredients and let sit for 2 hours, stirring occasionally

Coconut Chia Pudding – *from Liquid Raw*

1 young Thai coconut

2 tbsp. chia seeds

-Cut open the coconut and pour the water from the coconut into a large glass. Place 6 ounces of coconut water into a mixing bowl and add the chia seeds (you can drink any remaining coconut water). Mix the coconut water and chia seeds together, making sure that the seeds are thoroughly coated. Let soak for about 20 minutes, stirring occasionally to prevent clumping. Then scrape all the meat loose inside the coconut, but leave it in the coconut. Pour the coco-chia concoction back into the coconut. Chill and serve cool

-You can also add flavors such as vanilla, nutmeg, chai, or chopped banana and strawberry.

Healthy Cookies – *this recipe was taken from a Facebook post on "Way2aBetterYou". I haven't tried it yet, but it sound divine!*

2 cups Oats

3 mashed, ripe bananas

¼ cup almond milk (great time to try to make some yourself!)

1/3 cup apple juice

1 tsp. vanilla extract

1 tsp. cinnamon

½ cup raisins (optional)

-Mix all ingredients in a bowl. Drop by spoonful on a parchment paper lined cookie sheet and bake at 350° for 15-20 minutes. Enjoy!

Freckled Blonde Truffle – *from www.YoungAndRaw.com This recipe and the picture looked SO good that I had to share! These guys are free of gluten, refined sugars, and bad fats. They are also full of nutrients & fiber, can sustain your blood sugar and can even be eaten for breakfast!*

¼ cup honey

¼ cup organic, unrefined coconut oil

½ cup finely shredded organic raw dried coconut

½ cup raw organic cashews

¼ tsp ground vanilla or alcohol free liquid vanilla

3-4 tablespoons chia seeds

Pinch of Himalayan salt

-Place coconut and cashews in Vita-Mix (or other high speed blender or even a food processor) and blend until you reach flour-like consistency (about 10 seconds). Place in bowl. Melt coconut oil over a double boiler until liquid. Add honey, oil, vanilla, chia seeds and sea salt to bowl and mix until well combined, scraping sides a couple times. Chill in refrigerator for 45 mins. Once chilled, scoop by teaspoonfuls and roll into balls. Chill again for at least 10 minutes. Keep refrigerated until ready to eat. They can also be frozen.

Raw, Vegan Coconut Vanilla Yogurt – *from www.YoungAndRaw.com If you are trying to decrease or cut dairy completely out, this is one recipe that you should try. It's full of coconut goodness and it has lots of beneficial bacteria that are so very healing to your body. Best part is that you make it yourself!! So very empowering!*

2 cups coconut meat

1 tablespoon coconut kefir

1 tsp. dairy free probiotics (look for LIVE CULTURES)

1 tsp. vanilla bean

½ cup raw coconut water

-Blend all ingredients in your blender until creamy and smooth with no chunks left over. Pour into a glass jar and cover with a mesh fabric (like cheesecloth or thin dish towel) and elastic or nylon. Leave out in room temperature for 12 hours and then pop your jar in the fridge again for 1 day. Once the process is done, you should have a sour, tangy smell and taste (like yogurt). It's ready to eat!

-Option: you can add other ingredients like walnuts, almonds, dates, seeds or fresh fruit to give it a bit of variety. Play with your food!!

Candied Walnuts (iv) These can be used as a snack alone or they can be added to salads for added texture, nutrients, and sweetness

    4 cups raw walnut halves, toasted and skins removed

    ¼ cup EVOO

    ¼ cup agave nectar

    ¼ cup organic raw cane sugar

-In a large bowl, combine the walnuts with the EVOO and stir until thoroughly coated. Add the agave nectar and stir until thoroughly coated, then add sugar and stir until thoroughly coated. Warm a large cast-iron skillet to medium-high. Add the walnuts, scraping the bowl to remove everything, and stir constantly until the walnuts are fragrant and most of the liquid has evaporated (about 1 ½ minutes). Transfer to parchment paper and quickly spread out, separating them with two forks. Set aside to cool.

Minimalist Survival Snack Mix (iv) I saw this in Bryant Terry's book and thought it was a GREAT idea. When you are on-the-go and need a delicious, quick, healthy snack this is IT! Perfect blend of salty/sweet, crunchy/chewy, fruity/nutty.

    2 cups raw walnut halves (toasted if you'd like)

    1 ½ cups Thompson raisins

-Put both ingredients into a container, seal tightly, and mix thoroughly.

Let food be thy medicine and medicine be thy food.
– Hippocrates, Father of Modern Medicine

CHAPTER 14

A Final Word
Cß ßƆ

Every day, be better than the day before: You are only in competition with yourself – Facebook meme

Now that you've decided what your goals are, you've chosen the areas you want to work on, you've planned your strategy and you've begun the mental work to see it all through; it's time to set it all in motion.

Know that you can do it. Your greatest ally in achieving your goals is consistency. As long as you have a plan, you stick to it and you make changes or modifications as needed, you are bound to meet your short, medium and long term goals

Be like water – Bruce Lee

Know that it is probably not going to be easy. Doing most things that mean the most and are against the norm usually are not. It may never get easier, but I assure you that as you continue, you will become stronger and stronger. Eventually, you'll look back and see that you've come farther than you realize. Let that motivate you. Allow that realization to propel you forward.

Continue to monitor your progress, but don't beat yourself up when your progress seems to stall. It's ok. Keep persevering and modifying. Don't give up.

Finally, never, EVER compare yourself to anyone. Your journey is your journey. It's not like anyone else's. It's your race. It'll be your victory. You are a WINNER!!

It never gets easier, you just get better!!

CHAPTER 15

Additional Resources

I have tried many of the resources listed on these pages, but not all of them. When downloading any apps, be mindful of any permissions you are granting the company that developed it. As with everything else presented in this book, these are just used to give you a basic guide, some ideas. Begin to explore resources that you find work best for you in your Journey to Wellness and Improved Health.

The books that I've listed are geared towards vegetarian, vegan, or raw vegan food preparations. Know that I am by no means trying to convert the masses into raw vegans or even vegetarians. I'm not even a vegetarian (at least not most of the time). What I have found with these books is that they give me ideas on ways to cook a variety of meals that I may not have considered in the past. They help pull me out of my comfort zone and into exploring new foods and new ways of preparing familiar foods. Try them out for yourself. Broaden your food horizons while you grow stronger and healthier!

BOOKS

I absolutely LOVE books!! Often to a fault. I've had to clear out my bookcases several time in the last couple years because there were too many books on the shelves to keep up with. Here are just a few of my favorites, or those that are on my 'wish list', that I think would be great references for you. Happy reading!

The Vegan Soulfood Guide to the Galaxy by Afya Ibomu

Vegan Soulfood Kitchen by Bryant Terry

Afro-Vegan by Bryant Terry

The Beauty Detox Solution by Kimberly Snyder, C.N.

8 Weeks to Women's Wellness by Dr. Marianne Marchese

Liquid Raw by Lisa Montgomery

The Raw Truth: The Recipe for Reversing Diabetes by Kirt Tyson, N.M.D.

The Juicing Bible by Pat Crocker

Raw Food Real World: 100 Recipes to Get the Glow by Matthew Kenney and Sarma Melngailis

Raw: The UNcookbook by Juliano

The Anti-inflammatory Diet and Recipe Book by Jessica K. Black, N.D.

Eat Right 4 Your Type by Peter D'Adamo

Raw Foods for Busy People by Jordan Maerin

Tissue Cleansing Through Bowel Movement by Bernard Jensen, D.C., PhD

Water & Salt: The Essence of Life by Dr. med. Barbara Hendel, Peter Ferreira

Choose Your Foods: Like Your Life Depends on Them by Coleen Huber, N.M.D.

The Body Ecology Diet: Recovering Your Health and Rebuilding Your Immunity by Donna Gates

Cultured Food for Life: How to Make and Serve Delicious Probiotic Foods for Better Health and Wellness by Donna Schwenk

Ultimate Recipe e-book by Health-e-Solutions www.HealthESolutions.com

- This e-book contains recipes that are geared towards type 1 and 2 diabetics, but anyone can eat them. This family has tested the recipes on their children (they have two Type 1 diabetic boys) and with other children and found that they don't raise the blood sugars, no matter how much is eaten. I've tasted the foods they've prepared, and even prepared some myself, and let me tell you… they are TERRIFIC!!

Age Less, Live More: Achieving Health and Vitality at 107 and Beyond by Bernando LaPallo

- This book, though it has no recipes, is definitely one you should reference if you want to know how to live a long, healthy life. Mr. LaPallo wrote the book when he was 107 years old. I first met him when he was 109… and on a book signing tour. AMAZING right??!! Well, he is now 112 years old and still going strong. As a healthy, vibrant, independent elder with a terrific memory, a great sense of humor and fabulous health, I trust whatever he has to say about whatever he's saying. If you ever have an opportunity to listen to him speak or sit and have a conversation with him, you should take advantage of it. He's a joy to talk and listen to. If nothing else, at least go to YouTube and check out some of the videos of him speaking. He won't disappoint!

Earthing: The most important Healthy Discovery Ever? By Ober, Sinatra, and Zucker

- Here is a book that can teach you more about the benefits of Earthing and give you some ways that you can become more grounded in your own life.

APPS

On laughter

- Best Laugh Sounds by Starbranches (the best one that I've tried so far)
- I Am Laughing by Dimitris Van Leusden (second best that I've tried)
- Laugh Sounds by Apps4Mobile
- Laughing Sounds by Soda Pop
- Baby Sounds by BlackBeltStudio

On Bowel Movement

- Poop Log by Kefsco – Helps you track your BMs so that you can begin to see patterns and improvements over time
- Fiber Tracker by Kellogg Company – Helps you keep track of the amount of fiber you've eaten each day.

On Breathing and Relaxation

- Peaceful Breathing Lite by Steven Yi
- Anti-Stress Exercise by Quo?te Developers
- Breathing for Life
- Breathe 2 Relax by T2
- Take a Break from Stress by Meditation Oasis
- Meditation Helper by Multiordinal Limited
- Meditation Music by Pragar

On Water

- Water Your Body by NorthPark
- Drinking Water by Chickpin
- Water Reminder
- Drink Live Wallpaper by Happy, Inc

On Sleep

- Sleep App ~Dreamin~ by App Forge JP
- Nature Sounds Relax and Sleep by Zodinplex
- Nature Sounds to Sleep by Desenvdroid

- iHome Sleep by IHOME

On Food

- My Diet Diary Calorie Counter by MedHelp
- Food Planner by MiniMobile
- Is It Vegan? by ConnerBurggraf
- HappyCow VeginOut Free by HappyCow.net
  - This is a great site to help you find vegetarian/vegan friendly restaurants and other businesses all over the world. Can definitely help you eat better while away from home.
- Dirty Dozen by Environmental Working Group
  - If you don't want to print out the dirty dozen list, you can always load the app on your phone and have it with you all the time. The beautiful part is that the app updates each year when the new list comes out. So you don't have to keep checking. Isn't that great?!

On Fun

- How to Make Origami by Mobilicos
- Kids Origami by Gloding Inc.
- Hula Hoop by Dannielle
  - This is FABULOUS! It's a FREE, virtual hula hoop app that you can use anywhere. All you have to do is "turn on the app, place the phone at your hips, listen to the music, and shake your hips to keep it going." I can't wait to try it for myself!

WEBSITES AND ORGANIZATIONS

On Health

- www.HealthESolutions.com

- o This family mainly focuses on health as it pertains to diabetics, but the information it contains can be applied to anyone. Lots of useful food and lifestyle suggestions. And LOADS of great recipes that promote health, an alkaline pH, and steady blood sugars.
- www.CulturedFoodLife.com
  - o This site focuses on probiotic rich foods, also known as 'cultured' or fermented foods. These foods can be a huge asset in helping you reach the level of health that you want to attain. "Dramatically improve your health by eating foods filled with dynamic probiotics that supercharge your body!"
- www.HealthyJourneys.com
  - o This site provides a lot of high quality guided meditation CDs that range in topic from depression to ADHD to PTSD and Self Esteem. Whatever mental, or even physical, hurdle you are trying to overcome there is a guided meditation/imagery CD that can help you through it!
- www.EWG.org
  - o The Environmental Working Group (EWG) is a public health and environment protection organization that works really hard at giving us information about our health and how it's being impacted by corporations and other organizations. If you have any questions about the health and safety of skin care products, sunscreen, food, cleaning products or some other thing then you absolutely want to check them out!
- www.StraightUpFood.com
  - o This blog site gives you a whole host of recipes and resources for eating plant-based and vegan meals. If you'd like to incorporate more variety into your diet and would especially like to eat more veggies, but don't want to rely on salads, I highly encourage this site!

On Laughter

- www.LaughterYogaUSA.com
- www.LaugherYoga.org
- www.LaughterYogaAmerica.com
- www.MeetUp.com →
    - search this site for laughter groups in your area. Many of groups the MeetUp groups are free to join.
- www.YouTube.com →
    - Enter "Laughter Yoga", "Laugh Therapy", or "Laughter in your search"

On Clearing Clutter

- www.TheMinimalists.com
    - This site will guide you on how to get rid of all the extra "stuff" that surrounds you. You may not want to become a minimalist, but you can definitely use the principles and begin to free yourself of the extra junk that may be weighing you down in life. Remember, by clearing the physical space around you, you are clearing the space within you.
- www.BecomingMinimalist.com
- www.FatSickAndNearlyDead.com
    - Read the site watch the movie to get great tips and recipes on juicing, cleansing and healing. Follow Joe Cross on his journey to wellness as he learned to get rid of his old habits, and the old gunk that was inside his body. Watch how he transforms himself and encourages others to do so as well.
- www.RebootWithJoe.com
    - This is the online community for the film "Fat, Sick, and Nearly Dead"
- www.AllAboutJuicing.com

- o Visit this site to learn more about juicing and to get some GREAT juicing recipes.
- www.WendyIdaFitness.com
  - o This is the website for the AGE-DEFYING Wendy Ida. You will not believe that this beautiful woman is 60+ years old. REALLY! The awesome part of her story (as though that's not good enough) is that she didn't start her journey to health, healing and wellness until she was in her 40s. Proves that it is NEVER too late to be well!

ARTICLES

- "Laughter Yoga: Can Happiness Heal?" by Catherine Pearson. www.HuffingtonPost.com/US/entry/1478960
- How to do Laughter Yoga, Step-by-Step. www.WikiHow.com/Do-laughter-yoga
- Poop Color Chart (Helps you understand how the color of your poop can indicate your current health level). www.DoctorOz.com/videos/Poop-Color-Chart
- Bristol Stool Scale (Gives you a guide on how to assess your health by the quality of your poop) www.Wikipedia.org/wili/Bristol_Stool_Scale
- The Perfect Poop http://LifeSpa.com/The-Perfect-Poop/#.UifEoLt5vNA
- "What your poop and pee are telling you about your body" blog by Kimberly Snyder. This also contains a cool chart that you can print out and use.

VIDEO

On "The Force!"

- Star Wars V: The Empire Strikes Back scene with Yoda and Luke Skywalker http://youtu.be/BQ4yd2W50No

APPENDIX A

Sleep Hygiene

Sleep Hygiene is merely another way of saying good sleep habits. There are many factors that can improve the quality of a person's sleep. These listed below are thought to be some that will help to enhance good sleeping. When this is done, these strategies can provide long term solutions to those that are having sleeping difficulties. Certain medications and supplements can help with insomnia, but these are only short term solutions. Developing good sleep habits with the tips listed below along with discovering the root cause of the insomnia is a much more viable option in curing sleeping difficulties. Remember that improving the quality of sleep may not happen overnight, but with consistency it can happen!

1. **BE ON TIME:** Get in the habit of going to bed and waking up at roughly the same time every day, even on the weekends and holidays. Train your body to know when to sleep and when to wake.

2. **BED FOR SLEEPING ONLY:** Begin to use the bed for sleep and sex only. Do everything else (reading, computer, TV, etc.) in another part of the home. Teach the body to relate the bed to those two activities only.

3. **DEVELOP A ROUTINE:** Create a ritual that leads to sleep. By making this a habitual routine performed every night, you can help train your body to wind down and relax your way to sleep. Ex: Last meal at 6p. Most lights out by 7:30p. Soothing music on by 8p. TV off by 9p. Relaxing bath by 9p. Breathing exercises by 9:30. In bed by 10p.

4. **DON'T WATCH THE CLOCK:** The more you focus on the clock, the more anxious you are likely to become about the amount of time you are not sleeping. The more you are likely to reinforce negative sleep habits. Relax and ignore the clock.

5. **EXERCISE REGULARLY:** Getting regular exercise will help to condition the body and keep/get you in good health. Remember

not to exercise less than 3 hours before bedtime. You don't want to over stimulate yourself and keep yourself awake. Morning exercise is generally best.

6. **NO CAFFIENE OR NICOTINE:** Try not to consume Nicotine (cigarettes) or Caffeine (coffee, chocolate, sodas, green tea, away some medications) products 4-6 hours before bed. These products act as stimulants and can keep you awake longer than you'd like.

7. **DON'T JUST LAY THERE:** If you find that you cannot sleep after 20 minutes, get up and do something else until you get sleepy. Leave the bedroom and do something that will make you sleepy or something boring. Try to turn on as few lights as possible and avoid doing anything that is stimulating or interesting. You don't want to wake yourself up more. Lay back down in few minutes when you get sleepy again.

8. **RELAX:** Do what you can to relax as much as possible. Take a relaxing bath. Do some breathing exercises. Meditate. Turn off the action suspense murder mystery thriller.

9. **MAKE IT DARK AND QUIET:** Make your room as dark and quiet as possible to decrease the amount of interruptions, even small ones that can wake you up.

10. **GET SOME SUN:** Getting regular exposure to natural light, esp. in the early afternoon, has been show to help improve nighttime sleep

11. **TOO FULL OR EMPTY:** Don't go to bed too full or too empty. Both can disrupt sleep

12. **NAPS:** If you find that napping during the day makes it harder to sleep, avoid them. Otherwise, take them as often as possible.

13. **CHECK THE TEMP:** Make sure the temperature is comfortable in your room.

14. **WRITE IT DOWN:** If you find your mind racing at night, write down all the things you're thinking on a notepad. This will free your mind and allow you to relax.

If you'd like a one-page copy of this handout, go to the 'resources' section of my website: www.DrTursha.com.

Dirty Dozen, Clean 15

Here is the list of the most heavily contaminated, chemically laden produce crops of 2013. By avoiding these 12 foods listed on the dirty dozen, you can avoid upwards of 75% of the chemicals that you would normally ingest. So, take this list with you when you go shopping and arm yourself with the knowledge that you are doing right by your body!

For a second year, the EWG (Environmental Working Group) has added "Plus" to the list making it 14 total foods on the list. The last two are notable mentions that you should also consider buying organic.

♀ Apple	♀ Peaches
♀ Celery	♀ Potatoes
♀ Cherry Tomatoes	♀ Spinach
♀ Cucumbers	♀ Strawberries
♀ Grapes	♀ Sweet Bell Peppers
♀ Hot Peppers	♀ + Kale / Collard Greens
♀ Nectarines – imported	♀ + Summer Squash

The clean 15 are those veggies and fruit that are the least contaminated. These are ok if you decide to eat them non-organic.

✓ Asparagus	✓ Mangos
✓ Avocados	✓ Mushrooms
✓ Cabbage	✓ Onions
✓ Cantaloupe	✓ Papayas
✓ Sweet Corn	✓ Pineapples
✓ Eggplant	✓ Sweet Peas – frozen
✓ Grapefruit	✓ Sweet Potatoes
✓ Kiwi	

If you'd like to print the *Dirty Dozen, Clean 15* information, you can go to EWG.org and get a wallet card, or download one from the "Resources" section of my website: www.DrTursha.com.

Practically Healthy

Please contact Dr. Turshá Hamilton's office if you'd like:

- ❖ To schedule an appointment
- ❖ To book Dr. Turshá for speaking engagements
- ❖ More information about Naturopathic Medicine
- ❖ To order more books, CDs, DVDs, and other products by Dr. Turshá

Current (and soon to be released) titles by Dr. Turshá include:

- ❖ *Practically Healthy: Step-by-Step Guide to Better Health*
- ❖ *Practically Healthy: Roadmap to Success (workbook)*
- ❖ *Practically Healthy: 52 weeks to Better Health (motivational health cards)*

Dr. Turshá Hamilton

www.DrTursha.com

Phone: 480.420.7499

Email: info@DrTursha.com

You can also connect with Dr. Turshá on Facebook, Twitter, YouTube, and Instagram: *@DrTursha*

www.ingramcontent.com/pod-product-compliance
Lightning Source LLC
Chambersburg PA
CBHW072152270326
41930CB00011B/2396